Quick Easy Meals

Grain Free Cooking and Lose the Belly Fat

Sara Lee and Janice Carter

Copyright © 2013 Sara Lee and Janice Carter
All rights reserved.

Table of Contents

INTRODUCTION 1

SECTION 1: BELLY FAT DIET 6

CHAPTER 1: WHAT IS THE BELLY FAT DIET? 8

The Secret Behind the Diet 8

How the Diet Works 9

CHAPTER 2: BENEFITS OF THE BELLY FAT DIET 11

CHAPTER 3: ESSENTIAL TIPS FOR SUCCESS ON THE BELLY MELT DIET 14

Helpful Diet Tips to Follow 14

Top Belly Fat Burning Foods 16

CHAPTER 4: BELLY MELTING BREAKFAST RECIPES 19

   Banana Walnut Breakfast Muffin Recipe 20
   Tomato Pesto Eggs Florentine Breakfast Recipe 22
   Pumpkin Pie Flavored Oatmeal Breakfast Recipe 24
   Delicious French Toast with Chocolate Breakfast Recipe 26
   Belly Melt Huevos Ranchero's Breakfast Recipe 28
   Belly Filling Parfait with Granola Breakfast Recipe 30
   Decadent Walnut Banana Pancakes Breakfast Recipe 31
   Pecan and Cranberry Scones Breakfast Recipe 33
   Nut and Fruit Oatmeal Breakfast Recipe 35

CHAPTER 5: GREAT LUNCH RECIPES TO HELP YOU LOSE BELLY FAT 37

   Easy Turkey Pita with Side Salad Lunch Recipe 38

Shrimp, Barley and Baby Green Salad Lunch Recipe 40
Rainbow Veggie, Soba Noodle and Chicken Salad Lunch Recipe................ 42
Mediterranean Style Wraps Lunch Recipe 44
Low Sugar Strawberry and Peanut Butter Wraps Lunch Recipe 46
Easy Whole Wheat Muffin Pizzas Lunch Recipe.. 48
Walnut and Radish Spinach Salad Lunch Recipe.. 50

CHAPTER 6: FLAT BELLY DIET DINNER RECIPES 52

Smoked Salmon Frittata Dinner Recipe 53
Chicken Breast with Almond Crust Dinner Recipe 55
Easy Belly Busting Slow Cooker Chili Dinner Recipe.................................. 57
Snow Peas and Steamed Gingered Salmon Dinner Recipe 59
Chicken Roulade Stuffed with Spinach Dinner Recipe 61
Easy Whole Wheat Veggie Pizza Recipe 64
Roasted Pepper and Portobello Mushroom Burgers Recipe 67
Pepper Steak Tacos Dinner Recipe.. 69
Belly Flattening Broccoli Rabe Sausage Penne Recipe............................... 72

CHAPTER 7: BELLY FLATTENING DRINK, SNACK AND DESSERT RECIPES 75

Ricotta and Citrus Cannoli Dessert Recipe.. 75
Tasty Strawberry Tropical Fruit Smoothie Recipe 77
Delicious Apple Yogurt Dessert Recipe.. 79
Mocha Protein Health Snack Bites Recipe 81
Delicious Peanut Butter Balls Recipe... 83

CHAPTER 8: YOUR 7 DAY BELLY FAT DIET MEAL PLAN 85

SECTION 2: GRAIN FREE COOKBOOK 90

GRAIN FREE COOKBOOK RECIPES................................ 96

Grain Free Breakfast Recipes 96
Vanilla Yogurt with Fruit Salad... 96
Oven Omelet.. 98
Sweet Potato Breakfast Casserole.. 99

Nutty Hash	100
Breakfast Burrito	103
Apple Sausage	104
Coffee Cake	106

Grain Free Snacks, Appetizers, and Desserts 108
Peanut Butter Cookies	108
Cajun Fries	110
Curry Pumpkin Seeds	112
Oatmeal Chocolate Chip Raisin Cookies	113
Classic No Bake Cookies	115
Banana Date Cookies	117
Ginger Cookies	118
Raisin Spice Nut Cake	120
Tortilla Chips	122

Grain Free Breads 124
Irish Soda Bread	124
Corn Bread	126
Herbed Parmesan Bread	127
Banana Bread	129
Sandwich Bread	131
Zucchini Bread	133

Grain Free Side Dish Recipes 134
Broccoli Quinoa Casserole	134
Savory Black Bean Salad	136
Shrimp Soup	138
Mushroom Broccoli Tofu Quinoa	140
California Black Beans	141
Stuffing	143
Kale Mango Salad	146

Grain Free Main Dish Recipes 148
Parmesan Mushrooms Quinoa	148
Meaty Red Beans and Rice	150
Fried Rice	152
Jambalaya	154
Stuffed Cabbage	156
Spicy Meatballs and Rice	158
Stuffed Peppers	160

Salmon and Rice 162
Seafood Gumbo 164
Chicken Salad 166
Chicken Curry 168
Californian Chicken Soup 170
Beef Stew 172
Baked Salmon 174
Dutch Oven Chili 176

5 DAY MEAL PLAN 178

Introduction

Does the prospect of dealing with your belly fat make you feel upset and intimidated? Is your doctor asking you to reduce your waistline, and along with it your risk of heart disease, high blood pressure and diabetes? If you answered yes to these questions, it might be time to have a serious look at your diet.

Too many people follow a diet that's heavy in processed grains like refined wheat flour, along with even more manufactured foods such as high fructose corn syrup. These foods might be very appealing; in fact, they're designed to make you want to keep eating more and more. They can really take a toll on your health, however. When you use these foods in your cooking, you increase the number of calories you take in on a day to day basis. You also raise the chance that those excess with convert to fat, especially potentially dangerous belly fat.

Even very fit people who care a lot about their bodies can experience this problem. You might exercise regularly and watch what you eat, but suffer from stubborn belly fat. You might also have health problems that make it harder to get through your day. Many of these issues are caused by or made worse by all the grains and processed grain products that most people consume every day.

You don't have to put up with it, however. There's no reason that you should have to suffer with stubborn belly fat or unpleasant health issues. Simply by changing the way you eat and relying on healthier foods, you'll be able to cut down that fat, improve your body, and get back to a more natural way of living. The process might take a little bit of time, but when it's done, you'll wonder how you ever lived the way you do now.

This book is designed to help you learn how to get rid of your belly fat, boost your metabolism, and take care of your body by eating healthy, wholesome foods. It includes all the information you need to know about targeting stubborn fat and changing your diet for the better. Plus, you'll also get a wide variety of delicious recipes that rely on healthy, fat-burning foods. You'll be surprised by how much of a difference this simple change can make.

When you start reading, you'll see that this cookbook has been divided into two distinct sections. The first one focuses on belly fat, the best way to get rid of it, and how to eat in order to achieve that. The second part is designed specifically for people who want to decrease their reliance on unhealthy processed grains, especially health-damaging modern wheat flours. Together, these sections will help you understand why you're suffering from this belly fat problem and how best to combat it.

You'll get access to a wide range of great recipes designed to help you melt off that stubborn fat and improve your health. Try out our banana walnut breakfast muffins, fat-burning Huevos Rancheros, or fruit and nut oatmeal in the morning. Take easy turkey pitas and side salads to lunch, then come home to smoked salmon frittata or slow-cooked chili dinners that will help you burn off the calories without relying on excessive amounts of modified corn starch or processed white flour. Check out drinks and desserts that will help you cut back on belly fat, too. You'll love sweet, satisfying peanut butter balls and tropical fruit smoothies.

Choosing a lower-calorie diet and focusing on monounsaturated fatty acids is often enough to help you reduce your belly fat problem, but for some of us a more serious approach is required. This is often the case for people who have developed belly fat problems because they metabolize modern wheat varieties in a detrimental way. It's also a common situation if you happen to have a wheat intolerance or a digestive and immune condition such as celiac disease. In these cases, it's usually time to cut out wheat, as well as other modern, processed grains that can contribute to an excess of belly fat and an increased risk of diseases.

The second part of this book is designed especially for people who suffer from this problem. If you have trouble getting rid of your belly fat by following the recipes in the first portion of the book, or if you're someone who has known or suspected issues with wheat, it might be time to look at a grain-free or wheat-free diet. This might seem very difficult in a society where almost every kind of food contains wheat or processed grains of some kind, but it is possible.

You simply need to be willing to do your own cooking and shop smart. The grain-free recipes in this book are designed to help you with this issue, providing plenty of options to help you improve your health and get your body back into condition. Try out a grain-free breakfast with apple sausage or nutty hash. Choose a savory snack of curried pumpkin seeds or have a classic no-bake cookie without the damaging wheat usually found in this recipe.

For lunch, experience shrimp soup or broccoli quinoa casserole. Accompany it with a side of wheat or grain-free bread. Have a dinner made with stuffed cabbage or peppers and fresh chicken salad. If you can tolerate some grains but can't handle wheat, consider meaty red beans and rice or jambalaya. Remember: you don't have to give up flavor just because you're trying to cut down belly fat and get rid of unhealthy grains on your diet!

This book is here to help anyone who has trouble with wheat-induced health problems or stubborn belly fat. It's ready to act as the catalyst for your new, healthier diet and better body. With 5-day meal plans for each section and plenty of delicious recipes, it's the perfect option for anyone who has trouble dealing with conventional foods. If you're ready to get rid of your belly fat, it's time to start cooking now.

Section 1: Belly Fat Diet

Even if you have lost weight and you have toned up your body, you may still be dealing with stubborn belly fat. Belly fat is difficult to lose. You may be working out and trying to eat right, but it may seem that your belly just refuses to get flatter. If this is a problem you are dealing with, the belly fat diet may be the right diet for your needs. This diet is specifically designed to help you lose belly fat now. The foods included in the diet help target belly fat, helping you finally get rid of that belly.

This book is packed with all the information you need to successfully follow the belly fat diet and lose belly fat now. You will find helpful information on the diet, the benefits of following this diet and more. As you get started on the diet, you can enjoy using some of the helpful tips provided to ensure you are successful when you begin using this diet. The best part of this book is the many powerful recipes that will help support your belly melt diet. You will not have to start searching for recipes that go with your new diet.

Recipes are included for every meal. Great breakfast recipes will help you start out your day the right way. Tasty lunch recipes will keep you fueled up during the day and help you avoid cravings. The dinner recipes included will help you enjoy tasty meals that even your family will enjoy and many of them are ready in only a short amount of time, allowing you to add healthy eating to your busy life. You may be surprised to find dessert and snack recipes as well. Enjoy a delicious dessert or snack without sabotaging your belly fat diet.

You can finally get rid of that belly you have had for so long. Use these tips and the delicious recipes and included and you will quickly be on your way to a flatter belly.

Chapter 1: What is the Belly Fat Diet?

What is the belly fat diet? Maybe you have heard about this diet but you are not quite sure what it is and how it works. Basically, the belly fat diet is a special diet that is designed to help you take off inches of belly fat. You will lose weight while you are on this diet. However, the important part to note is that you will be taking off belly fat, not just losing a few pounds. While every individual is difference, most people end up losing 12-15 pounds within a month when they follow this diet. Several inches of belly fat are usually lost as well. The great thing about the diet is that you will not have to do hundreds of crunches to enjoy a flatter belly.

The Secret Behind the Diet

There is one big secret behind the diet – MUFAs. What are MUFAs? They are monounsaturated fatty acids. These fatty acids work to eliminate belly fat and they also make you feel full. Not only will you melt away belly fat when adding MUFAs to your diet, but these fatty acids will keep you feeling satisfied, which can help keep you from overeating as well. MUFAs are plant based fats and they can be found in foods like olive oil, chocolate, seeds, avocados and nuts. To get the best results while on this diet, you should strive to get a serving of MUFAs with every meal that you eat.

Even though MUFAs are fatty acids, these are healthy fats. They will not clog up your arteries. Instead, they actually help to improve your health. Along with the emphasis on MUFAs, which is the big secret behind this diet, the diet also emphasizes eating key foods like whole grains, fish, veggies, fruits, legumes and olive oil. In fact, this diet includes foods that are often found within the Mediterranean approach to eating.

How the Diet Works

Now that you know the secret behind the diet, you may be wondering how the diet works. The diet focuses on eating about 1600 calories a day and also involves eating a serving of MUFAs with each meal that you eat. Of course, keep in mind that you can tailor the number of calories you take in to your gender, activity level and your age. The diet includes avoiding processed, high fat foods. While protein is an important part of each meal, the focus is on vegetables and fruits with each meal.

The great thing about this diet is that most people find it very easy to follow. While you will have to restrict your diet to some extent, you still are able to enjoy wonderful meals that include delicious dishes. Many of the recipes included with this diet are easy to prepare, which makes this diet easy to follow, even for individuals that are very busy. You will not have to worry about skimping on taste either. Enjoy chocolate dishes, veggie pizzas and other great recipes that are sure to keep your taste buds happy.

Chapter 2: Benefits of the Belly Fat Diet

Belly fat, while it can be unsightly, can actually have serious long term health consequences. While going on the belly fat diet can help you lose your belly and feel better about the way you look, the main benefits of losing belly fat are health benefits. Unfortunately, while belly fat can be so dangerous, it is also extremely difficult to lose. Going on the belly fat diet can help blast away that belly fat. While you may already be excited about trying this diet, here are a few of the top benefits you can enjoy with this diet, which may excite you even more.

Benefit #1 – Reduce the Risk of Diabetes and Heart Disease

One of the best benefits of going on the belly fat diet is that it can help to reduce your risk of diabetes and heart disease. Excess belly fat can drastically increase your risk of developing diseases like diabetes and heart disease. In fact, excess belly fat can be almost as dangerous as smoking when it comes to increasing your risk of diseases like heart disease. The great news is that you can eliminate belly fat as a major risk factor for diabetes and heart disease. By following the belly fat diet, you can reduce your belly fat and begin reducing your risk of dealing with diabetes or heart disease in the future. In fact, your overall health will be improved as you melt that belly fat away.

Benefit #2 – Keep Testosterone Levels Normal

Studies show that having too much belly fat may lead to a reduction in testosterone within the body. This is especially troublesome for men, although women have testosterone as well. Low testosterone in men often causes impotence and lack of libido. The good news is that losing that belly fat can help keep testosterone at normal levels. Eliminating belly fat naturally begins to bring up testosterone levels. Adding exercise to the belly fat diet will boost levels of testosterone even more.

Benefit #3 – Enjoy Better Sleep at Night

Newer research that was done by Johns Hopkins shows that those who have more belly fat may not sleep as well as those with little belly fat. Losing belly fat may actually improve sleep quality. The study showed that those who reduced abdominal fat actually improved their sleep quality assessment test scores. This is important, since lack of sleep can cause a range of different health problems, including heart disease, depression and more. Simply losing some belly fat may be enough to help you sleep better, avoiding chronic lack of sleep.

Benefit #4 – Feel Better About Yourself

Last, the belly fat diet can help you blast away that troublesome belly fat, which has the benefit of helping you feel better about yourself. You may have a negative self-image of yourself while you still have belly fat. Losing the belly fat can help you improve your self-image, becoming happier with the way you look and feel. You may also enjoy feeling satisfied and triumphant when you succeed at improving your body and your health with the belly fat diet.

Chapter 3: Essential Tips for Success on the Belly Melt Diet

As you begin your belly fat diet, you want to ensure that you are successful. It can be easy to let a busy life get you off track when you are on a diet or to fall back into old habits that sabotage your efforts. To help you make the most of this diet, we have put together some great diet tips that will boost your belly melting efforts. You will also find a closer look at some of the top belly fat burning foods that you can work to add to this diet on a regular basis. With this information to guide you, you will have no problem making this diet successful.

Helpful Diet Tips to Follow

While the belly fat diet focuses on reducing calories, adding MUFAs and eating wholesome foods, there are some other tips you can follow to make the most of this diet. To help you get better results as you work to lose that belly fat, here are some helpful diet tips you definitely want to follow as you go on the belly fat diet.

- **Tip #1 – Avoid Drinking Your Calories** – On the belly fat diet, you should be taking in about 1600 calories each day. One of your best tips for success is to avoid drinking your calories. You may be surprised to find that many tasty drinks like shakes, juices and some coffee beverages can have hundreds of calories in a single drink. This quickly takes a big bite out of the calories you are supposed to have each day. Another big problem is that most of the calories in these drinks come from sugar, which can actually make your body store more belly fat instead of losing it. Instead of drinking your calories, focus on drinking plenty of water. You can also drink black coffee and certain teas without adding calories to your diet. Making this one simple change to your diet as you take on the belly fat diet can make a huge difference and help you lose that belly fat faster.

- **Tip #2 – Stay Away From Anything Processed and Refined** – Another helpful diet tip to follow while you are on the belly melt diet is to stay away from anything that is processed and refined. Processed foods usually have their nutrients stripped away when they are refined. They may also include many additives and sugar. That added sugar can make you feel hungrier, lead to more fat storage and can increase the production of insulin within your body. Processed, refined foods will sabotage your belly fat diet. Stay away from them and you are sure to enjoy better results.

- **Tip #3 – Don't Be Afraid to Cheat Once a Week** – It can be difficult to stick to a new diet all the time, especially if you are craving a specific food that you cannot have on your new diet. To make sure you stick with this belly fat diet, do not be afraid to cheat once a week. On one day, allow yourself to have one dessert that you have been craving or let yourself eat one cheeseburger or a slice of pizza. Knowing that you can cheat once a week can help you stick to your diet during the rest of the week. Feeling deprived can make you fail at your diet. Instead of feeling deprived, remind yourself that once each week you can enjoy cheating for a meal. It will go a long way towards helping you stick with the belly fat diet as you blast that fat away for good.

Top Belly Fat Burning Foods

While MUFAs are one of the big secrets to this belly fat diet, there are many other great belly fat burning foods that you can add to your diet to help you melt that belly fat. Here is a look at some of the top belly fat burning foods you should be eating and information on why they help you eliminate belly fat.

- **Fruits Rich in Fiber** – It is important to have plenty of fruits in your diet, especially those that are rich in fiber. They help make sure you get all the vitamins and minerals that your body needs. Berries are particularly important, since they are high in antioxidants and will help blast away belly fat. Some of the other great fruits that you should eat while on this diet include papayas, oranges, watermelon, peaches, cantaloupes, apples and apricots. Just make sure you eat fruits raw instead of drinking fruit juices.

- **Fiber Rich Veggies** – Veggies are an important part of your belly fat diet and they help make sure your body is burning off fat effectively. Some of the best vegies include leafy greens like cabbage, kale, lettuces and spinach. Other great veggies include cucumbers, broccoli, tomatoes and zucchini. Veggies can be eaten in salads, added to soups, stir fried, steamed or added to other dishes. The great thing about fiber rich veggies is that they fill you up and help to fight off cravings, which helps make it easier to lose belly fat.

- **Eggs** – Eggs are a powerful belly fat burning food to eat while following the belly fat diet. They have important vitamins that help your body burn fat. Eggs also have a lot of protein, which keeps you feeling full as well. Poach eggs, scramble them or even eat them hard boiled. They make a great breakfast that will fuel you for your day and help boost your belly melting efforts.

- **Green Tea** – Adding green tea to your belly fat diet is a great idea for several reasons. First, it works by flushing toxins out of your body naturally, eliminating water retention and bloating. It also has compounds that are known to help with weight loss, giving your metabolism a boost. Add a bit of lemon juice and honey to the tea for a very low calorie drink that will help burn fat.

- **Beans** – Different types of beans are a great addition to your belly fat diet as well. Beans are very high in protein, which can help to blast away stomach fat. Some great beans to try include Edamame, garbanzo beans, chick peas, kidney beans and black beans. Of course, when you add beans to your diet, avoid consuming them in large amounts. Too many beans can lead to bloating and gas, which will make your belly feel bigger.

These are just a few of the excellent foods that should be included in your belly fat diet. Along with the addition of MUFAs, they can help to blast away belly fat, helping you to enjoy success as you take on this new diet plan.

Chapter 4: Belly Melting Breakfast Recipes

Breakfast is the most important meal of your day, especially when you are trying to lose belly fat. On the belly fat diet, you need to make sure you get a good breakfast in your stomach to keep you feeling full until lunch. These recipes are packed with protein, fiber and healthy fats, helping you feel satisfied while ensuring you enjoy what you're eating.

Banana Walnut Breakfast Muffin Recipe

These delicious muffins make any breakfast special, including all the flavors you'd expect to find in a banana split. The great thing about these muffins is that they are perfect for your belly fat diet too. Breakfast will almost feel like dessert when you make these muffins for breakfast. In fact, you may want to make a few extras and freeze them to enjoy at a later date.

What You'll Need:

¾ cup of mini chocolate chips, semisweet
1 ½ cups of walnuts, chopped
¼ cup of canola oil
1 banana, very ripe and mashed
½ cup of dark brown sugar, packed
1 ½ cups of all-purpose flour
1 large egg
¼ cup of Greek yogurt, plain
½ teaspoon of ground cinnamon
¼ cup of skim milk
1 teaspoon of vanilla
1 tablespoon of baking powder
½ teaspoon of salt

How to Make It:

Start by preheating the oven to 375F. Add muffin papers to a muffin pan or use cooking spray to prepare a 12 cup muffin pan.

Add a half cup of walnuts to a food processor, processing until you have a very find powder. Next, place the freshly ground walnuts, baking powder, salt, flour, cinnamon, and chocolate chips in a large mixing bowl. Mix and combine thoroughly.

In a medium sized mixing bowl, combine the milk, vanilla, oil, egg, brown sugar, banana and yogurt. Stir until the mixture becomes smooth. Combine the flour and banana mixtures together, combining well. Last, stir the last cup of chopped walnuts into the batter. The batter should be quite thick.

Fill each muffin cup with the batter until about ¾ of the way full. Place muffins in the oven, allowing to bake for about 15 minutes. Check muffins for doneness. If the tops lightly spring back when you touch them, they are done. Remove muffins from the oven. Allow to sit for a few minutes. Then, remove each muffin from the muffin tin, placing them on a rack to cool. Makes 12 muffins.

Tomato Pesto Eggs Florentine Breakfast Recipe

A recipe from Prevention.com inspires this tasty recipe. It is easy to make, even for those who have never poached eggs in the past. While this recipe is wonderful for any breakfast, it makes a wonderful dish to serve guests for a nice brunch. It offers a nice mixture of protein, carbs and veggies, getting you ready for your shape. The bit of vinegar added to the recipe helps the egg whites to keep their shape while cooking.

What You'll Need:

1/3 cup of Greek yogurt, fat free
4 large eggs
1 teaspoon of olive oil
1 teaspoon of vinegar
1 9-oz package of baby spinach, prewashed
2 English muffins, whole grain, split and then toasted
¼ cup of sun-dried tomato pesto
Ground black pepper, freshly ground
Pinch of salt

How to Make It:

In a large skillet, heat up the olive oil on medium heat. One oil is hot, add spinach to the pan, cooking it just until it wilts. In a small bowl, combine the sun-dried tomato pesto and the yogurt. Then, stir a ¼ cup of the mixture into the spinach, immediate removing the spinach from the heat. Cover the skillet, keeping the spinach warm.

Meanwhile, add about 1 inch of water to a medium saucepan, heating it up on medium heat until it begins to boil. Once it starts boiling, add the salt and vinegar, turning the heat down to low. Break an egg into a small cup, then gently place the egg in the hot water. Do the same thing with each egg. Cover the pan, allowing the water to simmer. Cooking for about 3-5 minutes, shaking from a couple times. Yolks should start thickening and whites should be set when the eggs are done.

One four warmed plates, place half of an English muffin. Place about ¼ of the spinach mixture over the muffin. With a slotted spoon, remove poached eggs, draining them and placing on top of the spinach. Add a tablespoon of the poaching water to the leftover yogurt mixture, stirring it until smooth. Spread the yogurt mixture over eggs. Top with a bit of freshly ground pepper and serve right away. Makes four servings.

Pumpkin Pie Flavored Oatmeal Breakfast Recipe

This is a delicious belly fat buster that tastes amazing. You get the wonderful taste of pumpkin pie while blasting away belly fat. You'll also find that this oatmeal recipe is very filling, helping you avoid cravings throughout your day. Serve up this oatmeal with about a cup of skim milk. This only makes a single serving, so you may want to double or quadruple the recipe if you need to make more.

What You'll Need:

1/3 cup of quick cooking oats
1 teaspoons of brown sugar
1 cup of water
¼ cup of canned pure pumpkin (not pumpkin pie filling)
Pinch of ground cloves
Pinch of nutmeg
Pinch of salt
¼ teaspoon of ground cinnamon
2 tablespoons of pecans, chopped and toasted

How to Make It:

Heat up the water in a medium saucepan. Heat until water is boiling. After water comes to a boil, add the quick oats and the salt to the pan. Allow to cook for about 90 seconds. In a small bowl, combine the pumpkin, brown sugar, cloves, nutmeg, cinnamon and pecans. Reduce the heat of the oatmeal, once on low, stir the pumpkin pecan mixture into the oatmeal. Serve with skim milk. Makes a single serving.

Delicious French Toast with Chocolate Breakfast Recipe

If you have a bit of extra time on the weekend, this recipe is sure to be a hit with the family while going along with your belly fat diet. The great thing about this wonderful French toast recipe is that it offers plenty of fiber and protein for breakfast, which helps to keep you feeling full. Add fruit on the side for a well-rounded breakfast that you're sure to enjoy. After all, it's always nice to start the day with a bit of chocolate.

What You'll Need:

3 ounces of low fat cream cheese, softened
6 ounces of Italian bread, cut into 8 slices about a half inch thick
2 large egg whites
2 large eggs
4 ounces of semi-sweet chocolate, chopped finely
1 tablespoon of margarine, trans fat free
1 tablespoon of sugar
1 teaspoon of vanilla
1 teaspoon of orange zest, freshly grated
2 cups of fresh strawberries, sliced

How to Make It:

In a little bowl, combine the cream cheese and the chocolate together. In another bowl, combine the orange zest, sugar and strawberry slices.

On four slices of the Italian bread, spread a quarter of the cream cheese and chocolate mixture. Top each slice with another slice of bread, pressing slices together lightly.

In a medium sized bowl, combine the vanilla, egg whites and eggs. Whip lightly. Dip each side of the bread into the egg mixture, then setting the sandwich on a platter.

Place margarine in a large skillet, heating it on medium heat. When margarine is completely melted, place sandwiches into the skillet, cooking for about four minutes on each side. French toast should be cooked through and golden brown. Divide the fresh toast among four plates, topping the fresh toast with the strawberry mixture. Serve while hot. Makes four servings.

Belly Melt Huevos Ranchero's Breakfast Recipe

When you try this delicious breakfast recipe, you'll be surprised at all the flavor. It includes plenty of veggies and wonderful herbs add tons of flavor. The eggs give you plenty of protein, while you get your monounsaturated fats from the avocado that is included. If you like a little more kick when you eat your eggs, try adding just a bit of hot pepper sauce to the eggs when you eat them.

What You'll Need:

4 scallions, thinly sliced
1 teaspoon of ground cumin
2 cloves of garlic, minced
4 tablespoons of salsa
1 cup of avocado, sliced
½ cup of chicken broth, reduced-sodium
1 can of pink beans, no salt added, drained and rinsed
1 red bell pepper, sliced into thin strips
4 tablespoons of Greek yogurt, fat free
4 eggs
8 six-inch corn tortillas, toasted

How to Make It:

Begin heating a 10-inch skillet on medium heat. Place cumin in the pan, allowing to cook until it becomes fragrant. Only cook for about 30 seconds, stirring from time to time. Place the garlic, bell pepper, beans, broth and scallions in the skillet with the cumin. Bring the mixture to a boil, then reduce heat, allowing the mixture to simmer. Simmer for about eight minutes, ensuring that the vegetables become very tender and most of the chicken broth evaporates. Use a spoon to smash up the beans, making a thick, lumpy mixture.

With the back of a wooden spoon, make four different indentations in the mixture. Break an egg into a cup, pouring carefully into one of the indentations. Do the same thing with the rest of the eggs. Cover the skillet and allow eggs to cook for 8-10 minutes, ensuring that eggs are done to your taste.

Separate the mixture into four equal parts, ensuring each part has one egg. Place on four plates. Place slices of avocado around the beans. Use the salsa and yogurt to top the dish. Serve up with the toasted tortillas while hot. Makes four servings.

Belly Filling Parfait with Granola Breakfast Recipe

Not only is this parfait a delicious treat, but it is good for you to. You can make it in no time, which makes it great for busy mornings. It also looks elegant, which means you can serve this healthy breakfast up to guests and they'll never know how healthy it really is for them.

What You'll Need:

1 cup of raspberries
1 ½ cups of Granola
1 large banana, sliced
1 small 5.3 ounce container of Greek yogurt, fat free

How to Make It:

Place a small amount of granola in the bottom of a tall glass or parfait cup. Top with granola. Add fruit on top of granola. Repeat layers until the glass is full. Do the same thing in the second glass. Makes two servings, but it's easy to double the recipe to make more.

Decadent Walnut Banana Pancakes Breakfast Recipe

These pancakes are sensational and they'll help you work on gaining a flat belly too. You get a nice combination of crunchy and sweet with the walnuts and honey included in the recipe. The walnuts also add healthy, belly blasting fats to the recipe as well. This recipe includes plenty of fiber too, which means you'll stay feeling full longer. Serve with berries on the side for the perfect breakfast.

What You'll Need:

¼ cup of water
1 tablespoon of canola oil
½ cup of fresh raspberries
1 1/3 pancake mix, trans fat free
1 egg
1 teaspoon of vanilla
1 cup of buttermilk, low fat
¼ teaspoon of ground cinnamon
1 large banana, cut into very thin slices

1/3 cup of honey
1 tablespoon of water
½ cup of chopped walnuts

How to Make It:

In a large mixing bowl, combine the cinnamon and pancake mix. In a smaller bowl, combine the vanilla, egg, oil, buttermilk and water. Whisk the wet ingredients into the dry ingredients, stirring well until you have a smooth mixture. Fold the slices of banana into the pancake batter, setting to the side.

In a small bowl, combine the water, honey and walnuts.

Take a large nonstick skillet, coating it well with cooking spray. Place on medium heat and warm. Once the skillet is hot, begin adding batter by the ¼ cupful, cooking in batches. Pancakes should cook for about 2 minutes on each side, or until they become browned lightly.

Serve up pancakes, dividing among four separate plates. While hot, top with the walnut and honey mixture. Serve the raspberries on the side. Makes four servings.

Pecan and Cranberry Scones Breakfast Recipe

When you want a nice treat for breakfast, these scones are the perfect option. You can easily make a nice batch of the scones at the beginning of the week, storing them in the freezer so you can enjoy them all week. In fact, they are great if you need to grab your breakfast when you're headed out the door. The pecans add the monounsaturated fat to the recipe, helping it blast away your belly fat while enjoying a delicious breakfast.

What You'll Need:

1 ¼ cup of vanilla yogurt, low fat
1 cup of chopped pecans
2/3 cup of sweetened, dried cranberries
2 tablespoons of canola oil
2 cups of whole wheat pastry flour
½ teaspoon of baking soda
1 teaspoon of orange zest, freshly grated
½ teaspoon of salt
2 teaspoons of baking powder

How to Make It:

Preheat oven to 400F.

Coat a 9-inch round baking dish with some nonstick cooking spray.

In a large mixing bowl, mix together the baking powder, salt, baking soda, pecans and flour. In a smaller bowl, combine the orange zest, oil and yogurt. In the middle of the flour mixture, create a well, pouring the yogurt mixture into the well, as well as the cranberries. Stir the mixture until ingredients are blended.

Press the batter into the pan that has been prepared with cooking spray. Use a knife to score the dough, making eight triangles. Bake the scones for about 20-25 minutes. To check for doneness, insert a toothpick into the center. It should come out clean if the scones are done. Makes eight servings.

Nut and Fruit Oatmeal Breakfast Recipe

You probably already know how great oatmeal is for your heart. However, you may be unaware of how great it is for flattening your belly. This oatmeal recipe combines various nuts and fruits, adding plenty of flavor and great healthy fats that work to help you slim down that belly. You'll love the flavor of this oatmeal and you'll be surprised to find that it keeps you feeling full until lunch, so you may not even need a midmorning snack anymore.

What You'll Need:

½ cup of sweetened, dried cranberries
1 ¼ cup of rolled, old-fashioned oats
¼ cup of golden raisins
1 Granny Smith apple
1 cup of water
½ cup of walnuts, chopped
2 ½ cups of skim milk, divided

How to Make It:

Begin by washing the apple. Once washed, core the apple and then cut apple into ¼-inch chunks.

In a large saucepan, add 1 ½ cup of milk and the cup of water, bringing it to a boil with high heat. Stir in the oats, adding a pinch of salt if you desire. Heat should be reduced to low, allowing the oats to simmer for 3-4 minutes as the oats soften. Stir regularly.

Add the chopped apple to the oats. Cover the pan, allowing the oatmeal to simmer for about 3-4 more minutes. Oats should be slightly crisp, yet tender. Add raisins and cranberries. Remove the oatmeal from the heat, covering again and allowing it to stand for 1-2 minutes or until completely softened.

Scoop out oatmeal, dividing it up among four medium size bowls. Top each bowl of oatmeal with a ½ teaspoon of brown sugar and two tablespoons of the chopped walnuts. Add ¼ cup of the leftover skim milk to each bowl. Serve immediately. Makes four servings.

Chapter 5: Great Lunch Recipes to Help You Lose Belly Fat

It's important to eat a good lunch, since it will keep you from eating unhealthy snacks between lunch and dinner. Salads are always a great option for lunch and you'll find plenty of great salad recipes that fit in with your belly fat diet. Enjoy many tasty flavors while working to eliminate more belly fat. Try mixing up these recipes so you don't end up eating a salad every day, ensuring you don't get bored of salads.

Easy Turkey Pita with Side Salad Lunch Recipe

When you need a quick and easy lunch, this recipe is the perfect choice. The turkey offers plenty of great lean protein, plus, the veggies are great for helping you get that flat belly you desire. The olive oil in the side salad is a healthy, fat fighting, monounsaturated fat and the unique extras like the hearts of palm make sure you won't be bored with this salad.

What You'll Need:

Pita

1/8 cup of sprouts
¼ cup of baby spinach
4 ounces of turkey
1 whole wheat pita, small
4 small slices of tomato
1 teaspoon of Dijon mustard

Side Salad

½ cup of hearts of palm
1 cup of romaine lettuce, chopped
½ cup of red pepper, chopped
1 teaspoon of olive oil

½ cup of cucumber, chopped

How to Make It:

Cut the whole wheat pita in half. Spread insides of the pita with the mustard. Add slices of turkey to each half of the pita. Top with the sprouts, tomato slices and spinach.

Wash all the vegetables for the salad. Chop the romaine, peppers, cucumbers and cut up the hearts of palm into smaller pieces if needed. Toss all salad ingredients together. Drizzle the salad with the olive oil.

Makes a single serving.

Shrimp, Barley and Baby Green Salad Lunch Recipe

The curry powder and turmeric add a delicious flavor to this recipe, making it a salad that won't make you bored. The shrimp adds plenty of healthy protein to the salad without adding a lot of calories. The wide variety of vegetables makes sure you get plenty of crunch when you eat this salad, while you'll get some healthy fat from the pumpkin seeds added to the mix.

What You'll Need:

1 cup of barley
¼ cup of fresh basil, chopped
1 tablespoons of vegetable oil
3 cups of water
1 pound of shrimp, peeled, deveined and cooked
½ cup of cucumber, peeled and chopped
1 teaspoon of curry powder
1 tablespoons of lime juice, freshly squeezed
1 clove of garlic, minced
¾ cup of pumpkin seeds, toasted
1 ½ cups of tomatoes, diced and seeded
½ teaspoon of turmeric
2 teaspoons of jalapeno chili pepper, seeded and finely chopped

12 cups of baby greens
½ cup of green bell pepper, chopped
¼ teaspoon of salt
¼ cup of lemon juice

How to Make It:

Bring the water, turmeric and curry to a boil in a large saucepan. Once water is boiling, add the barley to the water. Cover the pan, reducing the heat and allowing to simmer. Allow barley to cook for approximately 40-45 minutes, until the barley becomes tender and the water has been absorbed. Remove barley from the heat.

While barley is cooking, whisk the oil, garlic, lime juice, lemon juice, salt and chili pepper together. Add the cucumber, tomatoes, shrimp, barley and bell pepper to the dressing mixture. Toss well to coat evenly.

On six plates, place two cups of the baby greens on each plate. Divide up the shrimp salad, adding salad on top of the bed of greens. Top with the pumpkin seeds and basil. Makes six servings.

Rainbow Veggie, Soba Noodle and Chicken Salad Lunch Recipe

The soba noodles, which can be substituted with whole wheat spaghetti, adds a nice amount of fiber to this salad. You'll get plenty of veggies from the peppers, snow peas and carrots. The avocado offers the monounsaturated fats you need in this meal. The soy sauce, pepper flakes, peanut oil and ginger really add a nice flavor to this salad. The bit of honey keeps the pucker factor under control.

What You'll Need:

2 tablespoons of lime juice, freshly squeezed
2 red bell peppers, seeded and sliced thinly
1 tablespoon of fresh ginger, grated
¼ cup of fresh cilantro, chopped coarsely
8 ounces of dry soba noodles or the same amount of whole wheat spaghetti
¼ teaspoon of red pepper flakes
2 cups of fresh snow peas, julienned
1 ½ cups of avocado, diced
2 tablespoons of honey
2 tablespoons of soy sauce, reduced sodium
2 tablespoons of peanut oil
1 cup of carrots, grated

2 cups of cooked chicken, shredded
2 tablespoons of rice wine vinegar

How to Make It:

Cook the soba noodles or spaghetti noodles according to the directions on the package. Once noodles are done cooking, drain well and then rinse with some cold water to ensure they stop cooking. Set noodles to the side.

Whisk the lime juice, ginger, soy sauce, vinegar, pepper flakes and honey together in a large bowl. Add the peanut oil in a steady stream while whisking the mixture. After dressing is well mixed, fold the bell peppers, avocado, noodles, cilantro, snow peas, carrots and chicken into the dressing. Serve immediately or chill and serve later. Makes six servings.

Mediterranean Style Wraps Lunch Recipe

The olive tapenade that is used in these wraps is an excellent source of monounsaturated fats, boosting the belly busting power of these tasty wraps. The chickpeas offer great protein to the wraps, while you'll get plenty of crunch from the peppers, onions and greens. The lemon juice and goat cheese makes these wraps full of incredible flavor. Make them the night before and take them to work for a healthy lunch that will keep you from eating out and ruining your belly fat diet.

What You'll Need:

4 cups of salad greens of choice
½ of a small red onion, sliced thinly
½ cup of canned chickpeas, no salt added, drained and rinsed
½ cup of green olive tapenade
2 ounces of goat cheese, crumbled
2 tablespoons of lemon juice, freshly squeezed
½ cup of jarred roasted red peppers, drained, sliced and dried
4 whole wheat tortillas or wraps (8-inches)
½ cup of seedless cucumber, sliced thinly

How to Make It:

In a large bowl, mix the lemon juice and green olive tapenade together with a fork. Add the peppers, onion, cucumber, greens and chickpeas to the mix, tossing to ensure they are well mixed. Add the goat cheese to the bowl, tossing gently to avoid breaking up the cheese further.

Warm the tortillas or wraps according to the directions on the package. Place a quarter of the mixture on the bottom of one of the wraps, rolling up securely. Cut the wrap in half at an angle, using a toothpick to keep the wraps together. Do the same thing with each of the wraps. Makes four servings.

Low Sugar Strawberry and Peanut Butter Wraps Lunch Recipe

Peanut butter and jelly is a timeless classic that is a favorite among kids and adults alike. This recipe brings you all the flavor that comes with a peanut butter and jelly sandwich. However, since it uses fruit instead of jelly, you don't have to worry about a meal that includes a lot of unneeded sugar. Also, the wraps add plenty of fiber to the meal, helping you stay full throughout the afternoon. Make these wraps to take to work and make a few extras for the kids as well. Everyone is sure to enjoy these healthy wraps that also help to shrink your belly.

What You'll Need:

1 cup of strawberries, sliced
2 8-inch whole wheat tortillas
4 tablespoons of natural crunchy peanut butter, preferably unsalted

How to Make It:

Place the tortillas on a work area. Spread each tortilla with half of the peanut butter, spreading carefully to avoid tearing the tortilla with the nuts in the peanut butter. Cover each tortilla with half of the strawberry slices. Roll each tortilla up. Slice diagonally into three sections. Makes two servings.

Easy Whole Wheat Muffin Pizzas Lunch Recipe

Whole wheat English muffins are much better for you than white ones, offering more fiber and a low calorie count. If you enjoy pizza, this is a great way to enjoy some of the wonderful flavors of pizza while sticking to your belly fat diet. You'll get delicious cheeses, great flavor from the basil and plenty of belly fat fighting healthy fats from the black tapenade used on the pizzas. They are easy to make and ready in no time, meaning you'll have a nice weekend lunch ready in a flash.

What You'll Need:

1 tomato, cut up into eight slices
4 teaspoons of Parmesan cheese, grated
½ cup of black tapenade
8 basil leaves, fresh
1 cup of reduced fat mozzarella cheese, shredded
4 whole wheat English muffins, split in half

How to Make It:

Preheat oven to 400F.

After splitting the English muffins, toast them. Once toasted, each muffin half should be spread with about a tablespoon of the black tapenade. 1 tomato slice should go on each muffin half. Top the tomatoes with a ½ teaspoon of Parmesan cheese and about 2 tablespoons of the mozzarella.

Place each English muffin half on a baking sheet. Place pizzas in the oven, allowing to take for 6-8 minutes, ensuring that the cheese is well melted. Remove from the oven, topping with a leaf of basil before serving. Serve right away. Makes four servings. You can also make extras and store them in the fridge for a couple days. They make a great snack.

Walnut and Radish Spinach Salad Lunch Recipe

While the walnuts and olive oil add the important monounsaturated fats to this recipe, the baby spinach and radishes offer plenty of important nutrients for the body. The lemon juice, white wine vinegar and black pepper produce plenty of great flavor. Not only does this salad make a wonderful lunch recipe, but it's a nice side dish that can be served up with dinner as well.

What You'll Need:

4 medium sized radishes, sliced thinly
1 tablespoon of lemon juice, freshly squeezed
¼ cup of extra virgin olive oil
½ cup of walnuts, halved
2 teaspoons of white wine vinegar
5 ounces of baby spinach
Black pepper, freshly ground, to taste
Salt, to taste

How to Make It:

Whisk the vinegar and lemon juice together in a large bowl. Add pepper and salt to taste. Slowly pour in the olive oil, whisking continually.

Right before serving, toss the radishes and spinach with the dressing, coating greens completely. Divide up the salad among four different salad plates. Top the salad with walnuts. Serve right away. Makes four servings.

Chapter 6: Flat Belly Diet Dinner Recipes

Eating a good dinner will help you avoid those late night snack cravings, which can quickly sabotage your belly fat diet. All of these recipes include some form of monounsaturated fat, which helps to blast away that belly fat that you are working so hard to lose. You'll find great fish recipes, meatless recipes and more. Even if you need a dinner in a hurry, you'll find easy, fast recipes that allow you to eat a healthy dinner, even on your busiest days.

Smoked Salmon Frittata Dinner Recipe

It's always nice to have a breakfast style recipe for dinner. This dinner recipe makes use of eggs and salmon, ensuring you get plenty of protein. The salmon is full of healthy Omega-3s, which are important if you want to enjoy a flatter belly. The combination of protein and healthy fats help ensure you won't be reaching for a late night snack later in the evening.

What You'll Need:

4 eggs
6 egg whites
2 ounces of smoked salmon, thinly sliced and cut into pieces (about ½-inch wide)
6 scallions, trimmed and chopped coarsely
¼ cup of cold water
¾ cup of black olive tapenade
½ teaspoon of salt
1 ½ teaspoons of fresh tarragon, chopped
2 teaspoons of extra virgin olive oil
Black pepper, freshly ground

How to Make It:

Preheat oven to 350F.

On medium heat, heat up an 8-inch skillet that is ovenproof, heating on medium for about a minute. Place olive oil in the skillet, adding scallions to the oil. Sauté the scallions until they are soft, stirring regularly.

Whisk the tarragon, salt, egg whites, water and eggs together in a medium sized bowl. Add black pepper to taste. Pour the egg mixture into the skillet, topping with the pieces of salmon. Allow to cook for about two minutes, stirring from time to time, allowing eggs to set partially.

Place the skillet with the egg mixture into the oven, allowing to cook for 6-8 minutes. Eggs should be puffed, firm and golden brown on top. Remove the skillet from the oven. Release the frittata from the skillet with a spatula. Slide carefully onto a serving platter that has been warmed.

On six plates, spread about two tablespoons of the black olive tapenade. Top the tapenade with a slice of frittata. Eat immediately while hot. Makes six servings.

Chicken Breast with Almond Crust Dinner Recipe

Chicken packs a powerful protein punch, but it's lower in fat than certain other meats, as long as you don't use the skin. This recipe calls for skinless and boneless chicken breasts, so you don't have to worry about removing the skin. The almond crust makes the chicken something special and also keeps the inside from drying out while you cook it. Serve up with some tomatoes and cottage cheese on the side for a wonderful meal that will keep you feeling satisfied. Keep in mind, this recipe is only for a single serving, so if you're feeling a family or guests, you may need to make extra to fit your needs.

What You'll Need:

1 tablespoon of cornstarch
2 tablespoons of almonds, chopped finely
¼ cup of egg substitute, fat free
5 ounces of skinless, boneless chicken breast

How to Make It:

Sprinkle chicken breasts generously with cornstarch on both sides. After nicely coated with the cornstarch, dip the chicken breast into the egg substitute, ensuring it's well coated. After coated with the egg substitute, sprinkle the chopped almonds over the chicken on both sides.

Spray nonstick cooking spray on a nonstick skillet, heating it up on medium. Place chicken breast in the skilled, cooking for about five minutes per side until done. The thickest part of the chicken breast should reach 165 degrees F to make it safe to consume. Makes a single serving.

Easy Belly Busting Slow Cooker Chili Dinner Recipe

This chili recipe is so easy to make. Since you can put it in the slow cooker, it makes dinner so easy for busy individuals that want a meal that is ready to eat for dinner. With olive oil and avocados, you're getting the fat busting monounsaturated fats that you need. The chili beans add extra protein to the chili and instead of meat, soy crumbles are used, allowing you to enjoy a nice, meat-free dish from time to time.

What You'll Need:

1 can of chili beans (14 oz.), drained and rinsed
1 tablespoon of extra virgin olive oil
1 green bell pepper, seeded and then diced
Chili powder to taste
1 cup of avocado, chopped
1 can of whole tomatoes, salt free (28 oz.)
1 tablespoon of onion, minced
12 ounces of soy crumbles, fat free

How to Make It:

Combine the soy crumbles, onion, oil, chili powder, pepper, tomatoes and beans in a four quart slow cooker.

Cover the slow cooker, cooking on low for 8-10 hours or on high for 4-6 hours. Chili should be well thickened by the time it's done cooking. Scoop chili into four bowls. Top with avocado pieces and serve hot. Makes four servings.

Snow Peas and Steamed Gingered Salmon Dinner Recipe

Salmon is a great protein choice to eat while you are trying to slim down that belly. Not only does it provide a low calorie form of protein, but it also includes healthy fats that help to eliminate that belly fat. The sesame oil, lime juice, ginger, garlic and soy sauce all make a delicious glaze that provides the great flavor for this steamed salmon. Chopped avocado adds even more healthy fats to the meal and the snow peas round it out to be an easy meal that won't take long to fix for dinner.

What You'll Need:

1 clove of garlic, minced
1 cup of avocado, chopped
1 teaspoon of fresh ginger, grated
2 scallions, sliced thinly
1 tablespoon of lime juice, freshly squeezed
1 pound of trimmed snow peas
1 teaspoon of toasted sesame oil
2 teaspoons of soy sauce, reduced sodium
4 salmon fillets, skinless and about 1.5 inches thick

How to Make It:

Rub the garlic and ginger on the salmon fillets. Use nonstick cooking spray to coat a steaming basket. Place the salmon fillets into the basket. Bring about two inches of water to boiling in a large saucepan. Add the steamer basket to the pan, covering and allowing the salmon to steam for about 7-9 minutes.

While the salmon is steaming, whisk the soy sauce, scallions, oil and lime juice together in a small bowl, setting to the side for later.

Once the salmon has been steaming for 7-9 minutes, add the snow peas on top of the salmon in the steamer basket. Allow the peas and salmon to steam for another 4-5 minutes, making sure that salmon is well cooked and the peas are tender yet crispy.

On four plates, arrange snow peas to make a bed for the salmon. Top the snow peas with the salmon. Top each salmon fillet with some of the avocado pieces. Drizzle with the soy sauce mixture. Serve right away while hot. Makes four servings.

Chicken Roulade Stuffed with Spinach Dinner Recipe

Not only does this delicious chicken recipe taste amazing, but it looks great served up on dinner plates as well. It's easy enough to make for a family dinner at home. However, it's elegant enough to make for guests as well. Enjoy plenty of flavor with the red pepper flakes and the sun dried tomatoes. The spinach adds plenty of nutrition to this healthy dish as well.

What You'll Need:

2 teaspoons of olive oil
½ cup of dry white wine or chicken broth
¼ cup of onion, finely chopped
¼ cup of Parmesan cheese, grated
1 10oz package of frozen chopped spinach
1/3 teaspoon of red pepper flakes
2 tablespoons of dry packed sun dried tomatoes, chopped
1 clove of garlic, grated or crushed
4 chicken breast halves, carefully trimmed and pounded into very thin cutlets

How to Make It:

Make the frozen spinach according to the directions on the package. Once cooked, place spinach in a strainer, using a spoon to help press out the extra liquid. You should have about ½ cup of spinach left.

While spinach is cooking, place a teaspoon of the olive oil in a nonstick skillet, heating on medium heat. Add the garlic, onion, 1 tablespoon of water and the red pepper flakes to the skillet. Allow to cook until onion begins to sizzle. Reduce heat to low, covering and allowing to cook until the onion is softened, which should take about 2-4 minutes. Stir once while cooking.

When spinach is ready, stir the spinach, cheese and onion mixture together in a little bowl. Keep the skillet to the side to use later.

On the smooth side of the chicken cutlets, sprinkle with the tomatoes. Divide the spinach mixture, spreading it evenly on each cutlet. Leave about an inch at the narrow end without the spread. Roll up the chicken cutlets loosely, using a wooden toothpick to secure it.

Add the rest of the olive oil to the previously used skilled. Heat oil on medium heat, adding the chicken to the skillet, browning chicken on every side for about 10 minutes. Add the dry white wine to the skillet, covering the skillet and allowing the chicken to cook on low for another 7-8 minutes. Uncover the pan, moving chicken to a warm serving dish. Use foil to cover the chicken, keeping it warm until serving.

Bring the leftover juices in the skillet to a boil until you have a nice glaze. This should take approximately 4-5 minutes. Slice the chicken roulades diagonally into pieces about an inch thick. Drizzle with the glaze and then serve while warm. Makes four servings.

Easy Whole Wheat Veggie Pizza Recipe

As you work hard to lose belly fat, you still do not want to give up some of your favorite foods. The good news is that you can still enjoy having pizza while you are on the flat belly diet. This recipe makes use of many great veggies that will fill you up while allowing you to enjoy some pizza. The mixture of mozzarella cheese, Parmesan cheese, basil, mushrooms, peppers and pesto will provide you with plenty of great flavor as you enjoy this delicious pizza dish.

What You'll Need:

½ cup of finely sliced red onion
¾ cup of cherry tomatoes, quartered
¼ cup of sun-dried tomato pesto
2 tablespoons of Parmesan cheese, grated
2 teaspoons of olive oil
1 cup of button mushrooms, sliced
1 cup of sliced zucchini
½ cup of basil leaves, thinly sliced
1 cup of yellow or orange bell peppers, sliced thinly
1 whole wheat pizza crust, thin

How to Make It:

Begin by preheating the oven to 425F.

Work the whole wheat pizza crust out on the pizza pan, ensuring the entire pan is covered with the crust. Take the pesto and spread it out evenly over the crust. Place the peppers, onion, mushrooms and zucchini in a bowl. Pour in the olive oil. Toss the vegetables in the olive oil until they are coated.

Place veggies in a skillet heated over medium heat. Saute the vegetables for 5-8 minutes or until the veggies have turned soft and the liquid from the veggies has evaporated.

Sprinkle the cheeses over the crust, making sure the crust is covered evenly. Take the sautéed veggies and add them to the pizza crust on top of the cheese. Top the pizza with the tomato pieces.

Place the pizza in the oven, allowing to bake for 18-20 minutes. The crust should be baked throughout and should be crisped slightly on the bottom. Remove from the oven. While hot, sprinkle the pizza with the sliced basil leaves. Allow to stand for 5 minutes. Cut the pizza into quarters and then serve. Makes four servings.

Roasted Pepper and Portobello Mushroom Burgers Recipe

If you find yourself craving the delicious flavor of a burger while you are following the flat belly diet, you will definitely love this tasty recipe. You do not have to worry about the calories and fat that comes with beef, since no meat is used within this recipe. Portobello mushroom caps make up the burger part of the recipes and these mushrooms are full of rich, delicious flavor that will let you enjoy the flavor of a burger without all the fat and calories. The addition of roasted bell peppers and pesto really amp up the flavor, making this a burger that will make your taste buds sing while you enjoy working on a flatter belly.

What You'll Need:

2 roasted red bell pepper halves, jarred
4 leaves of frisee lettuce, or other lettuce you have on hand
4 small to medium Portobello mushroom caps, about 8 ounces
2 tablespoons of pesto, prepared
4 teaspoons of balsamic vinegar
2 whole wheat hamburger buns

How to Make It:

Over medium heat, preheat a large grill pan.

Place the Portobello mushroom caps on the grill pan, grilling them for four minutes on each side. While mushroom caps are cooking, continue to brush with the balsamic vinegar. When mushrooms are nearly done, warm the buns and the bell pepper halves on the grill pan too.

Spread half of the pesto on each of the hamburger buns. On the bottom of each bun, place 1 of the red pepper slices and two mushroom caps. Top with 2 pieces of the lettuce. If desired, add just a little bit more vinegar. Top with the top of the bun. Enjoy immediately. Makes two servings.

Pepper Steak Tacos Dinner Recipe

Eating lean protein and whole grains can help you enjoy flatter abs and this delicious recipe includes some of the best belly slimming ingredients to make a delicious dinner. The flank steak used within the recipe offers a lot of lean protein. You will get plenty of veggies in this dish as well, including bell peppers, corn, avocado, jalapenos and more. Enjoy making this recipe up for a nice dinner. You may even want to make some extras so you can take some to work for a nice, healthy lunch.

What You'll Need:

3 teaspoons of olive oil
½ cup of frozen or fresh corn kernels
¼ cup of Monterey Jack cheese, low fat, grated
2 cloves of garlic, crushed
1 lime, juiced + lime wedges when serving the dish
½ teaspoon of mild chili powder
¼ cup of salsa Verde
3 bell peppers, thinly sliced (1 orange, 1 red and 1 yellow)
1 teaspoon of kosher salt
½ red onion, thinly sliced
½ avocado, sliced
2 tablespoons of pickled jalapenos, sliced

1 pound of flank steak
Light sour cream to taste

How to Make It:

Mix together the lime juice, crushed garlic, chili powder and salt in a sealable plastic bag. Add the flank steak to the bag, shaking up so the marinade coats the steak. Place the marinating steak into the refrigerator for about 20-30 minutes, minimum.

While the steak is marinating, place a cast iron skillet on medium high heat until well heated. Add two teaspoons of the olive oil to the skillet. Place the bell peppers and red onion in the skillet, allowing to cook for about five minutes, tossing and stirring while cooking. Place the corn kernels in the skillet, continuing to cook the vegetables for about 3-4 more minutes or until the peppers become soft and slightly charred. When veggies are done cooking, place them in a medium bowl and place in the microwave to keep warm.

Use a paper towel to wipe out the skillet. Heat the skillet for a minute and then add in the leftover teaspoon of the olive oil. Take steak out of the marinade, using paper towels to pat it dry. Place the steak in the pan and cook over medium high heat for four minutes on each side.

Once the steak is done cooking, remove it from the pan and place on a cutting board. Allow the steak to rest for 5-7 minutes.

Use a sharp knife to slice the flank steak, cutting across the grain. Arrange the steak on a large platter with lime wedges and peppers. Warm tortillas and then begin making tacos. Place steak and peppers in the tortillas, adding avocado, cheese, jalapenos, salsa and the sour cream. Enjoy. Makes four servings.

Belly Flattening Broccoli Rabe Sausage Penne Recipe

Whole wheat pasta is a great addition to your belly fat diet. It fills you up but it does not spike blood sugar like white pasta does. Instead of using traditional, high fat sausages, this recipe uses turkey sausages, which offer a lot of protein without all the fat usually found in sausage. This recipe gets plenty of flavor from the crushed red pepper flakes, ricotta cheese and the Parmesan cheese. The great thing about this recipe is that you can have it ready in under a half hour, making it a quick, easy dinner to use during the week when you are really busy.

What You'll Need:

½ red onion, sliced thinly
12 ounces of whole wheat penne pasta
2 tablespoons of tomato paste
1 clove of garlic, thinly sliced
2 tablespoons of Parmesan, grated
1 medium bunch of broccoli rabe
2 Italian turkey sausages with the casings removed
¼ cup of ricotta cheese, part skim
Pinch of crushed red pepper flakes
1 tablespoon of extra virgin olive oil

How to Make It:

Fill a large pot with water, adding a bit of salt. Bring the water to a boil. Once boiling, add the broccoli rabe to the water, allowing it to cook for about 3-5 minutes. Remove broccoli rabe from the boiling water, placing it in a colander to drain and cool. Once you can handle it, chop it up into bite-size chunks.

Bring the same pot of water back to boiling. Place the whole wheat penne in the boiling water. Cook until it is al dente. Set aside ½ cup of the pasta water and then drain the penne pasta.

While the penne is cooking, place a large skillet over medium heat. Add the olive oil and allow it to heat up. Add the garlic, onion, red pepper flakes and sausages to the hot olive oil. Use a wooden spoon to break up the sausages. Cook the mixture until the sausages are well browned, which will take about eight minutes. Then, place the broccoli rabe into the pan with the sausage mixture, continuing to cook until the rabe becomes tender, about 2-3 more minutes.

Turn the heat under the skillet down to low. Place the drained pasta in the skillet with the sausage mixture.

Toss well to make sure all the ingredients are combined. If the mixture seems a bit dry, add a small amount of the reserved pasta water to the pan. Stir the Parmesan and ricotta cheeses into the pan, removing the pan from the heat and tossing again. Serve the pasta dish right away. Makes six servings.

Chapter 7: Belly Flattening Drink, Snack and Dessert Recipes

Ricotta and Citrus Cannoli Dessert Recipe

Just because you're following a belly fat diet doesn't mean that you have to skip out on a tasty dessert. This dessert will go well with your diet, helping you to achieve the flat belly you really want. Of course, you shouldn't overindulge on these delicious delicacies, but it's fine to enjoy one from time to time. It also makes a wonderful, belly friendly dessert to make if you're having guests for dinner. It goes wonderful with a few slices of banana and strawberries on the side.

What You'll Need:

1 tablespoon of orange zest, freshly grated
½ teaspoon of pure vanilla extract
1/3 cup of powdered sugar
3 cups of chocolate chips, semi-sweet, divided
16-ounces of ricotta cheese, fat free

1 teaspoon of lime zest, freshly grated
2 teaspoons of lemon zest, freshly grated
12 cannoli shells, large

How to Make It:

Combine the vanilla, orange zest, lime zest, lemon zest, powdered sugar and ricotta in a medium sized mixing bowl. Use an electric mixer to whip the mixture together until it becomes fluffy and very light. Fold 2 ½ cups of the chocolate chips into the ricotta mixture, saving the last ½ cup of chocolate chips for later.

Take cannoli shells, dividing up the filling evenly among the shells. Use a spoon to get the filling into the shells or you can pipe it in with a plastic bag that has the tip cut off. Melt the rest of the chocolate chips. Drizzle the chocolate on top of every cannoli. Allow chocolate to harden. Place in the refrigerator. Serve cannoli chilled. Makes 12 servings.

Tasty Strawberry Tropical Fruit Smoothie Recipe

Just a taste of this delicious smoothie is like being in paradise. Enjoy sipping on this drink while imagining you are far away on the beach. Not only does this smoothie taste amazing, but it is good for you. It will help you lose weight and flatten that belly, especially since it adds in some flaxseed oil to the mix. When you are craving something a bit sweet, this will help you fix that craving.

What You'll Need:

1 cup of vanilla yogurt, fat free
1 ½ cup of frozen peach slices
½ cup of mango nectar, chilled
1 cup of fresh strawberries, hulled and cut in half
2 tablespoons of flaxseed oil
1 tablespoon of frozen pineapple juice concentrate, thawed slightly

How to Make It:

In a large blender, place the yogurt, frozen peach slices, mango nectar, strawberries and the pineapple juice concentrate. Blend the ingredients until they become smooth and well combined. Once well blended, add the flaxseed oil to the blender, only blending enough to combine thoroughly.

Pour the blender contents into two large glasses. Add a strawberry half to each glass as a garnish. Enjoy the smoothie right away. Makes two servings.

Delicious Apple Yogurt Dessert Recipe

This wonderful apple yogurt dessert recipe allows you to enjoy something sweet without sabotaging your belly fat diet. You will get to enjoy all the flavors found in apple crisp without the high calories and fat that come with that tasty dessert. The addition of Greek yogurt makes sure you get plenty of protein while you enjoy a sweet treat. Make this for dessert after dinner or enjoy it as a sweet snack at any time of day.

What You'll Need:

2 tablespoons of apple sauce
¾ cup of plain Greek yogurt (or vanilla)
1 teaspoon of honey
Pinch of nutmeg
Pinch of cinnamon
1 Granny smith apple, cored, peeled and diced

How to Make It:

In a small bowl, mix together the apple sauce, honey and Greek yogurt. Stir in the diced apple. Top with a pinch of nutmeg and cinnamon. Mix everything together. Eat right away. Makes a single serving. You may want to double or triple the recipe if you want to serve this dish up to the family as a dessert.

Mocha Protein Health Snack Bites Recipe

If you find yourself craving some chocolate, these delicious mocha bits will help you to quash that craving. Not only will you get your chocolate hit, but you will also get some protein when you eat these bites as well. Keep a couple with you during the day for a tasty, protein rich snack that will keep you going and help you reduce other cravings. They are very easy to make and everyone is sure to enjoy them.

What You'll Need:

6 egg whites
1 teaspoon of coffee
¾ cup of oatmeal
2 granny smith apples, diced
¼ teaspoon of baking powder
1 scoop of chocolate protein shake powder
1 drop of vanilla extract
¼ cup of Quaker oats
2 tablespoons of apple sauce
1 teaspoon of honey
½ teaspoon of cinnamon

How to Make It:

Preheat the oven to 350F.

Place the egg whites, coffee, oatmeal, baking powder, protein shake powder, vanilla, Quaker oats, apple sauce, honey and cinnamon in a blender. Blend the ingredients together until you have a thick mixture. Pour the mixture into a large bowl. Add the diced apples to the mixture, using a spoon to mix the apples into the mix.

Spray an 8x8 inch baking dish with cooking spray. Pour the mixture into the baking dish. Place the baking dish in the oven, baking the mixture for about 25-30 minutes. Remove from the oven and allow to cool.

Once the bites have cooled, cut into eight equal pieces. Makes eight servings. Store bites in a container for up to 3 days.

Delicious Peanut Butter Balls Recipe

Not only do these peanut butter balls make a wonderful dessert or snack, but they pack a great protein punch as well, which can help you meet your flat belly goals. They are really easy to make and once you make up the balls, you'll have a quick snack or dessert that you can grab when you have a craving. Since they have a lot of protein, they will help you stay full and enable you to stick with your belly fat diet.

What You'll Need:

1 teaspoon of vanilla extract
1 cup of Stevia, Splenda or another sugar alternative
4 scoops of vanilla or chocolate protein powder
1 cup of peanut butter, sugar free

How to Make It:

Place the vanilla, sugar alternative, protein powder and peanut butter in a medium bowl. Mix the ingredients together until they are well combined. After the ingredients are well mixed, take tablespoon sized portions and roll them into bowls, placing on wax paper. Once all the balls are rolled, place in the refrigerator until the peanut butter balls are set. Store in an airtight container.

Chapter 8: Your 7 Day Belly Fat Diet Meal Plan

Getting started on a new diet is always difficult, especially when you are trying to figure out how to plan meals so you stick with it. To make it easier for you to stay on your belly fat diet, you can follow this 7-day belly fat diet meal plan. It provides great meals for breakfast, lunch and dinner, as well as some great snack ideas. Follow this plan for the first few days to get you started. Once you are used to the diet, you can mix and match recipes within the book as you continue working to lose that belly fat.

Day 1:

Breakfast: Tomato Pesto Eggs Florentine Breakfast Recipe

Lunch: Easy Whole Wheat Muffin Pizzas Lunch Recipe

Dinner: Chicken Breast with Almond Crust Dinner Recipe

Snack: Mocha Protein Health Snack Bites Recipe

Day 2:

Breakfast: Banana Walnut Breakfast Muffin Recipe

Lunch: Mediterranean Style Wraps Lunch Recipe

Dinner: Snow Peas and Steamed Gingered Salmon Dinner Recipe

Snack: Tasty Strawberry Tropical Fruit Smoothie Recipe

Day 3:

Breakfast: Delicious French Toast with Chocolate Breakfast Recipe

Lunch: Walnut and Radish Spinach Salad Lunch Recipe

Dinner: Smoked Salmon Frittata Dinner Recipe

Snack: Delicious Peanut Butter Balls Recipe

Day 4:

Breakfast: Pumpkin Pie Flavored Oatmeal Breakfast Recipe

Lunch: Low Sugar Strawberry and Peanut Butter Wraps Lunch Recipe

Dinner: Easy Belly Busting Slow Cooker Chili Dinner Recipe

Snack:

Day 5:

Breakfast: Belly Filling Parfait with Granola Breakfast Recipe

Lunch: Easy Turkey Pita with Side Salad Lunch Recipe

Dinner: Chicken Roulade Stuffed with Spinach Dinner Recipe

Snack: Ricotta and Citrus Cannoli Dessert Recipe

Day 6:

Breakfast: Belly Melt Huevos Ranchero's Breakfast Recipe

Lunch: Rainbow Veggie, Soba Noodle and Chicken Salad Lunch Recipe

Dinner: Roasted Pepper and Portobello Mushroom Burgers Recipe

Snack: Leftover Delicious Peanut Butter Balls

Day 7:

Breakfast: Pecan and Cranberry Scones Breakfast Recipe

Lunch: Shrimp, Barley and Baby Green Salad Lunch Recipe

Dinner: Easy Whole Wheat Veggie Pizza Recipe

Snack: Delicious Apple Yogurt Dessert Recipe

Section 2: Grain Free Cookbook

Normally, when people talk about going grain free they mean particularly wheat free. Wheat is found in so many food products today, especially in processed foods. However, the there is a rise in the number of people who experience health issues if they consume wheat, and in particular, the gluten part of the wheat. With the rise of wheat or gluten intolerances and allergies, the need for more alternatives for food has surfaced. First, let's talk about the health issues consuming wheat may cause.

Health Issues From Consuming Wheat

Wheat has a high glycemic index level. This means it converts to "sugar" easily in the body, which in turns converts to excessive weight gain and fat. People wanting to lose weight may find if they avoid wheat, they lose the weight easier.

Allergies to wheat can cause symptoms of IBS or irritable bowel syndrome. Other issues that may show up are migraine headaches, asthma irritations, fatigue, skin issues, and yeast infections. Sometimes people will have one or more of these symptoms and after going off the wheat will find relief. If you have any of these symptoms, you may ask your healthcare provider about having an allergy test done to see if it is caused by wheat. Or try the diet and see if you have relief.

Autism patients may show improvement if they go on a gluten free diet. For parents of autistic children, this is good news, as it may provide some help in treatment. Again, ask the healthcare provider about this possibility.

Some people may have difficulties in the absorption of minerals if they consume wheat. This may be why they show the above symptoms. Certainly, it is best for the body if it is able to absorb all the nutrients from the foods we eat. Going on a grain free diet allows the body to have a chance to absorb all the nutrients from nutritious foods.

Tips for a Grain Free Diet

If you have studied the grain free diet you may have run across a diet called the Paleo Diet. This is a diet believed eaten by our Stone Age ancestors. The main component of the diet is the absence of grains. This grain free cookbook is not the Paleo Diet, because the recipes here do include foods on the "avoid" list for the Paleo Diet, but it is interesting that it is also a popular diet that works that does not include grains. Our Stone Age ancestors were a healthy bunch, living to ripe old ages (older than we do) and without many of the health ailments we suffer.

In addition to the recipes included in this book, there are ways to avoid grains if you stop and think about it. The first thing you should do is plan your meals. You may want to vary your meals, by cooking stuff that is not included in this book. That is okay, you stay "grain free" if you simply avoid grains. Here are some tips:

For breakfast, look at the recipes provided here and include healthy portions of eggs. Eggs are so versatile; you can fry them, scramble them, poach them, and boil them. And in addition to all of that, you can serve them with sautéed vegetables, cheese, or even with a slice of grain free bread or coffee cake. Eggs are a good source of protein and they give you a good energy boost to start your day.

Think outside the box of wheat products. If you love spaghetti, instead of reaching for the wheat laden noodles, grab a couple of zucchinis and slice them lengthwise into "noodles." Pour a bit of spaghetti sauce over and try the Herbed Parmesan Bread and you will have a delicious Italian meal. Carrots can be done this way as well.

Are you a pizza lover? Try making a flat omelet (there is those eggs again, versatile, aren't they?) and spread pizza sauce and toppings. You will not miss the wheat crust, because the flavors of the all the pizza will over power the egg. Try it you will be surprised!

If you do not have any bread ready for a sandwich, make a lettuce roll. Put all the items you would in your sandwich on a big lettuce leaf, roll it up and eat it. It will taste great and you will remain grain free. You can do the same thing with hamburgers, sloppy Joes, or any kind of sandwich meal.

Get to eating more soups and salads and forget sandwiches, if you are addicted to breads. Soups and salads are very satisfying and a lot more nutritious than 2 slices of wheat bread. Of course, if you are a hardcore sandwich lover, there is a recipe for wheat free sandwich bread in this book.

What About All the Hype About How It Is Healthy to Eat Whole Grains

It is true, if you research about going grain free you will find as many articles about how healthy whole grains are, and it can get confusing. The only way to know for sure if you have a gluten or wheat intolerance is either to have allergy tests performed, or try an elimination diet.

An elimination diet may be helpful in pinpointing whether or not certain foods actually cause issues or not. It takes a little while to figure this out though, you cannot just avoid a certain food for a day and figure it out. For one thing, it takes the body a couple of days to even a week or two for the side effects of certain foods to leave the body. With this in mind, if you do choose to try an elimination diet, you need to stick with it for at least three weeks to see the full effects.

If it is wheat foods that concern you and you wish to try the elimination diet to see if that indeed is the culprit to your health issues, this grain free cookbook is your perfect companion. Each recipe is completely wheat grain free, so you can easily plan three weeks' worth of meals to find out if wheat is your problem.

A Good Way to Get a Healthy Whole Grain

A food called quinoa acts as a grain, but in truth is even healthier than whole wheat. This food has been consumed for thousands of years. Quinoa is one of the "super foods" that packs a load of nutrition. What makes quinoa so wonderful is how it can be used in recipes. A few recipes within this book that contains quinoa and it is an excellent replacement for whole grains. The good thing about quinoa is that there are hardly any instances of people with "quinoa allergies" or "quinoa intolerances."

Suggestions for using this Grain Free Cookbook

The recipes within this book contain healthy whole ingredients. But the recipe by itself is not meant to be the only thing consumed. Include other foods with your meals. For example, eat salads with lunch and supper, steam vegetables for side dishes. Feel free to add to these recipes to enhance them. The recipes within this book may be similar to others, however each one is meant to be a part of the grain free diet and offers a variety in choices.

Grain Free Cookbook Recipes

Grain Free Breakfast Recipes

Vanilla Yogurt with Fruit Salad

A refreshing breakfast, and highly nutritious, you cannot go wrong with this delicious fruit salad with a sweet vanilla yogurt.

What You'll Need:

1 banana (just ripe, sliced)
1 bunch of seedless grapes (green, halved)
2 cups of yogurt (plain)
2 cups of strawberries (tops cut, halved)
1 cup of blueberries
1 cup of raspberries
2 tablespoons of honey
1 tablespoon of orange juice
1/2 teaspoon of vanilla extract

How to Make It:

Mix the 2 cups of plain yogurt with the 2 tablespoons of honey and the 1/2 teaspoon of vanilla extract with a whisk. In a separate bowl, add the banana slices and the tablespoon of orange juice. Add the 2 cups of halved strawberries, cup of blueberries, cup of raspberries, and the bunch of seedless halved green grapes and toss with the banana slices. Divide the fruit into 6 individual bowls, top with the sweetened vanilla yogurt.

Makes 6 servings.

Oven Omelet

This is an easy omelet to make because you do not have to worry with flipping it in the pan. Just mix the ingredients and put in a baking dish and an hour later have a hot fresh omelet.

What You'll Need:

16 eggs
2 cups of milk
2 cups of cheddar cheese (sharp, shredded)
3/4 cup of turkey ham (cubed)
6 scallions (chopped)
salt and pepper

How to Make It:

Prep: Preheat the oven to 350 degrees Fahrenheit. Spray a 13x9 in baking dish with cooking spray.

Add the 16 eggs to a bowl and stir with a whisk, making sure to break each yolk. Pour in the 2 cups of milk and continue whisking. Add the 2 cups of shredded sharp cheddar cheese, 3/4 cup of cubed turkey ham, 6 chopped scallions, and season with salt and pepper. Stir to combine. Pour into the greased baking dish. Bake for about 47 minutes. Insert a knife in the middle, the omelet is cooked when the knife comes out clean. Allow to cool for ten minutes before serving.

Makes 12 servings.

Addition: Add 1/2 cup of finely chopped bell peppers to make it a western omelet.

Sweet Potato Breakfast Casserole

This is a different twist on a breakfast casserole with the addition of the sweet potato.

What You'll Need:

1 dozen eggs
1 pound of turkey breakfast sausage
2 1/2 cups of spinach (baby, chopped)
2 cups of sweet potatoes (diced)
1 scallion (diced)
salt and pepper
canola oil

How to Make It:

Prep: Preheat the oven to 375 degrees Fahrenheit. Spray a 9x13 inch baking dish with cooking spray.

First, add a little canola oil to a skillet and turn to medium high. Cook the pound of turkey breakfast sausage until browned. Add a little more canola oil if needed to cook the 2 cups of diced sweet potatoes until tender. Next, place the tender diced sweet potatoes in a large bowl. Toss in the 2 1/2 cups of chopped baby spinach, and the diced scallion. Add the cooked sausage and the salt and pepper to taste to the vegetables. Place into the greased baking dish. Next, crack the dozen eggs in a large bowl and whisk until smooth. Salt and pepper the eggs if desired. Pour the eggs over the sausage and vegetables. Bake for about 27 minutes. Remove from oven and sit for 10 minutes before cutting and serving.

Makes 8 servings.

Nutty Hash

This chunky hash is full of the goodness of apples, squash and pecans and makes a hearty and satisfying breakfast.

What You'll Need:

2 cups of squash (butternut, diced)
1 1/2 cups of apples (tart, diced)
1/2 cup of pecans (chopped)
1/4 cup of scallions (chopped)
1/4 cup of onions (chopped)
2 tablespoons of olive oil
1/2 teaspoon of salt
1/2 teaspoon of black pepper

How to Make It:
Preheat the oven to low broil.

Heat a skillet on the stove on medium heat. Place the 2 cups of diced butternut squash onto a lined baking sheet. Broil and flip the squash every 3 minutes until it just starts to brown. Take out of the oven, turn oven off. Drizzle the 2 tablespoons of olive oil into the hot skillet. Add the 1/4 cup of chopped onions and sauté. Put the sautéed onions in a bowl. Add the 1/2 cup of chopped pecans to the skillet and heat through. Next add the 2 cups of browned squash, 1 1/2 cups of diced tart apples, the cooked onions to the heated pecans and stir a couple of times to combine, then allow to sit so it will soften. After a couple of minutes, flip and stir it to release the steam. Once browned to your liking, remove from heat. Sprinkle the 1/4 cup of chopped scallions over the top and sprinkle the 1/2 teaspoons of salt and pepper. Serve and enjoy.

Makes 4 servings.

Breakfast Burrito

Here is a delicious breakfast burrito made with turkey ham and the spiciness of salsa.

What You'll Need:

8 eggs
4 slices of ham (big enough slices to wrap with)
1/4 cup of spinach (chopped, baby)
1/4 cup of black olives (chopped)
1/4 cup of bell pepper (chopped, your color choice)
1/4 cup of tomato (chopped)
Salsa
Guacamole
Cilantro (for garnish)
Canola oil

How to Make It:

First, heat a skillet to medium high. Drizzle enough canola oil into a skillet to sauté the 1/4 cups of chopped baby spinach, black olives, bell pepper, and tomato. Whisk the 8 eggs in a bowl and pour over the cooking vegetable until scrambled. Even spoon the eggs onto each slice of turkey ham. Roll the turkey ham to make a meat burrito. Place back in the skillet, carefully rolling to heat and slightly brown the ham. Serve on a plate with salsa and guacamole. Garnish with a sprig of cilantro.

Makes 4 servings.

Apple Sausage

This is actually a very different sausage, pork-free and made with chicken and apples.

What You'll Need:

1 pound of ground chicken
1 large apple (peeled, cored, grated)
1 egg
1 teaspoon of salt
1/2 teaspoon of basil (dried)
1/2 teaspoon of cumin (ground)
1/2 teaspoon of marjoram (dried)
1/2 teaspoon of oregano (dried)
1/2 teaspoon of sage (dried)
1/2 teaspoon of thyme (dried)
1/4 teaspoon of black pepper

How to Make It:

Prep: Preheat the oven to 350 degrees Fahrenheit. Line a baking sheet with parchment.

Beat the egg first, then add it to the 1 pound of ground chicken, 1 large apple (peeled, cored, grated), 1 teaspoon of salt, 1/2 teaspoon of basil (dried), 1/2 teaspoon of cumin (ground), 1/2 teaspoon of marjoram (dried), 1/2 teaspoon of oregano (dried), 1/2 teaspoon of sage (dried), 1/2 teaspoon of thyme (dried), and 1/4 teaspoon of black pepper. With hands, mix the ingredients. Form into 18 patties and place on the baking sheets, sides not touching. Bake for 10 minutes and flip, then bake another 10 minutes.

Makes 9 two-patty servings.

Coffee Cake

There is nothing more mouthwatering than the smell of delicious coffee cake baking first thing in the morning.

What You'll Need:

4 eggs
1 cup of pecans (chopped)
3/4 cup of arrowroot flour
3/4 cup of coconut flour (sifted plus 1 teaspoon)
1/2 cup of almond milk
1/2 cup of honey (plus 2 tablespoons)
1/2 cup of butter (1/4 cup melted and 1/4 cup softened)
2 teaspoons of baking powder
1 1/2 teaspoons of cinnamon (ground)
1/2 teaspoon of salt

How to Make It:

Prep: Preheat oven to 350 degrees Fahrenheit. Spray an 8x8 inch baking pan with cooking spray.

In a bowl, beat the 4 eggs then combine with the 1/2 cup of almond milk, 1/2 cup of honey, and the 1/4 cup of melted butter. In a separate bowl, combine the 3/4 cup of arrowroot flour, 3/4 cup of sifted coconut flour, 2 teaspoons of baking powder, and the 1/2 teaspoon of salt. Gradually add the dry ingredients into the batter, stirring to combine.

In another separate bowl, make the streusel. Combine the 1 cup of chopped pecans, 1/4 cup of softened butter, 2 tablespoons of honey, and the 1 1/2 teaspoons of ground cinnamon.

Pour half of the batter into the greased baking dish. Sprinkle half of the streusel. Pour the remaining batter over the streusel and sprinkle the remaining streusel on top. Bake until a knife inserted in the middle comes out clean, about half an hour.

Makes 6 to 8 servings.

Grain Free Snacks, Appetizers, and Desserts

Peanut Butter Cookies

A very chewy and delicious peanut butter cookie, you will enjoy eating.

What You'll Need:

2 cups of peanut butter
2 cups of sugar (granulated, plus extra for dusting)
2 eggs (slightly beaten)
2 teaspoons of vanilla extract
Coarse salt granules

How to Make It:

Prep: Preheat the oven to 350 degrees Fahrenheit.

Combine the 2 cups of peanut butter, 2 cups of granulated sugar, 2 beaten eggs, and the 2 teaspoons of vanilla in a bowl. Drop by the tablespoonful's onto a baking sheet (ungreased), and flatten crisscross with a fork. Sprinkle extra sugar and coarse salt granules over the top. Bake for about ten minutes until the cooked turn a golden brown. Keep an eye, oven baking times vary. Let sit in baking sheet for 2 minutes before carefully removing with a spatula to a wire rack for continued cooling.

Makes 3 dozen.

Cajun Fries

This is a nutritious snack but tastes like it's forbidden because of its wonderful spiciness. Enjoy!

What You'll Need:

10 carrots (peeled, cut into thin sticks)
1 tablespoon of olive oil
1/4 teaspoon of cayenne pepper (OR use a Cajun seasoning)
Salt and Pepper
Dipping sauce

How to Make It:

Prep: Preheat the oven to 450 degrees Fahrenheit. Spray a baking sheet with cooking spray.

Put the carrot sticks in a large zipper bag and drizzle the tablespoon of olive oil, 1/4 teaspoon of cayenne pepper and some salt and pepper into the bag. Zip and shake to coat each carrot stick. Next, place the carrot sticks onto the baking sheet and place in the oven for about 15 minutes. Turn each "fry" over and continue to bake for another 15 minutes. Delicious served warm.

Dipping sauce: Try your favorite dipping sauce for French fries or chicken strips. For example, ranch dressing, honey mustard, or ketchup.

Curry Pumpkin Seeds

For those who love curry seasoning and pumpkin seeds you will love this snack!

What You'll Need:

2 cups of pumpkin seeds
2 egg whites
4 teaspoons of curry powder
salt

How to Make It:

Prep: Preheat the oven to 375 degrees Fahrenheit. Place a piece of foil over a baking sheet.

Whisk the 2 egg whites together with the 4 teaspoons of curry powder and as much salt as you'd like. Place the 2 cups of pumpkin seeds into a large bowl with a lid. Pour the seasoned egg whites over the pumpkin seeds, place the lid on the bowl and shake, to evenly coat all the pumpkin seeds. Spread out over the foil in a single layer on the baking sheet. Bake until the seeds turn a golden brown, about 12 minutes. You can store in a zipper back and sprinkle more curry powder and salt as desired.

Oatmeal Chocolate Chip Raisin Cookies

These cookies are chewy, spicy, and perfect for a snack or treat.

What You'll Need:

4 1/2 cups of oats (old fashioned)
1 cup of butter (softened)
3/4 cup of sugar (granulated)
3/4 cup of chocolate chips (your favorite kind)
3/4 cup of raisins
1/2 cup of brown sugar (light, packed)
2 eggs
2 tablespoons of cornstarch
2 teaspoons of vanilla extract
1 1/2 teaspoons of cinnamon (ground)
1 teaspoon of baking powder
1/2 teaspoon of salt

How to Make It:

Prep: Preheat the oven to 350 degrees Fahrenheit. Line a cookie sheet with parchment.

Add 1 1/2 cups of the old fashioned oats to a food processor or blender and process to a fine meal. Stir in the 2 tablespoons of cornstarch, teaspoon of baking powder, and the 1/2 teaspoon of salt.

In a separate bowl, combine the cup of softened butter with the 3/4 cup of granulated sugar and the 1/2 cup of packed light brown sugar. Use an electric beater to mix for about a minute. Add the 2 eggs and the 2 teaspoons of vanilla extract and beat for another minute. Turn the beater to low and gradually add the prepared 1 1/2 cup of oats, for about a minute. Scrap the beaters. Fold in the remaining 3 cups of oats, 3/4 cup of chocolate chips, and the 3/4 cup of raisins.

Drop a large heaping tablespoon of dough onto the lined cookie sheet, leaving a 2 inch space between the cookies. Bake for about 15 minutes, until golden brown. Let the cookies cool for two minutes before carefully removing to a wire rack.

Makes 3 dozen cookies.

Classic No Bake Cookies

This is a classic favorite, like a candy bar in the shape of a cookie!

What You'll Need:

3 cups of oats (quick cooking)
2 cups of sugar (granulated)
1/2 cup of peanut butter
1/2 cup of butter
1/2 cup of milk
3 tablespoons of cocoa powder (unsweetened)
1 teaspoon of vanilla extract
pinch of salt

How to Make It:

Place a saucepan on high heat and add the 2 cups of granulated sugar, 1/2 cup of butter, 1/2 cup of milk, and the 3 tablespoons of unsweetened cocoa powder. Stir continually until the mixture boils and boil while stirring for 60 seconds. Turn the heat off but keep on the burner. Add the 3 cups of quick cooking oats, 1/2 cup of peanut butter, and the teaspoon of vanilla extract, stirring until the peanut butter melts and all combines. Drop by spoonful's onto waxed paper to form into cookies and cool. Store uneaten portions in the refrigerator.

Makes 4 dozen.

Banana Date Cookies

This delicious snack is as nutritious as it is tasty.

What You'll Need:

3 bananas (ripe)
2 cups of oats (rolled)
1 cup of dates (pitted, chopped)
1/3 cup of canola oil
1 teaspoon of vanilla extract

How to Make It:

Prep: Preheat the oven to 350 degrees Fahrenheit.

First, peel the bananas and mash them in a bowl. Add the 2 cups of rolled oats, 1 cup of pitted and chopped dates, 1/3 cup of canola oil, and the 1 teaspoon of vanilla extract. Mix and set aside for 15 minutes. Drop by spoonful's onto an ungreased baking sheet. Bake until light golden brown, about 20 minutes. Cool before serving.

Makes 3 dozen.

Ginger Cookies

These are like ginger snaps only they have coconut and cinnamon.

What You'll Need:

2 cups of almond flour
1/2 cup of coconut (grated)
1/3 cup of honey
4 tablespoons of butter (melted)
1 teaspoon of ginger (ground)
1/2 teaspoon of cinnamon (ground)
1/4 teaspoon of baking soda
1/8 teaspoon of salt

How to Make It:

Prep: Preheat oven to 300 degrees Fahrenheit. Spray a cookie sheet with butter flavored cooking spray.

In a bowl, add the 1/2 cup of coconut , 1/3 cup of honey, 4 tablespoons of butter,
1 teaspoon of ginger, and 1/2 teaspoon of cinnamon and combine by stirring. In a separate bowl combine the 2 cups of almond flour with the 1/4 teaspoon of baking soda and 1/8 teaspoon of salt. Stir the dry ingredients

into the batter. Shape into palm sized balls (about an inch in diameter) and place on the greased cookie sheet. Bake until golden brown for about 12 minutes.

Makes 2 to 3 dozen cookies (depending on how big you make them).

Raisin Spice Nut Cake

A delicious spice cake chocked full of walnuts and raisins.

What You'll Need:

2 1/2 cups of almond flour
2 eggs (beaten)
1/2 cup of yogurt (plain)
1/2 cup of walnuts (chopped)
1/3 cup of raisins
1/3 cup of honey
4 tablespoons of butter (melted)
1 teaspoon of vanilla extract
1 teaspoon of cinnamon (ground)
1 teaspoon of allspice
1/2 teaspoon of nutmeg (ground)
1/2 teaspoon of baking soda
1/4 teaspoon of salt
1/4 teaspoon of cloves (ground)

How to Make It:

Prep: Preheat the oven to 300 degrees Fahrenheit. Spray an 8x8 inch baking pan with cooking spray. Combine the 2 beaten eggs with the 1/2 cup of plain yogurt, 1/3 cup of honey, 4 tablespoons of melted butter, and the teaspoon of vanilla extract. In a separate bowl, combine the 2 1/2 cups of almond flour with the teaspoons of ground cinnamon, allspice, 1/2 teaspoons of ground nutmeg, baking soda, 1/4 teaspoons of salt and ground cloves. Gradually add the dry ingredients into the batter. Fold in the 1/2 cup of chopped walnuts and the 1/3 cup of raisins. Pour the batter into the prepared 8x8 inch baking pan and bake until the top is golden brown, about half an hour.

Makes 6 to 8 servings.

Tortilla Chips

These "tortilla" chips can go either salty or sweet, whichever your tastes happens to be when you make them.

What You'll Need:

8 egg whites
1/2 cup of water
1/4 cup of coconut flour (raw)
1/4 teaspoon of baking powder
Butter
(salt OR cinnamon and sugar)

How to Make It:

Combine the 1/4 cup of raw coconut flour with the 1/4 teaspoon of baking powder. Add the 8 egg whites and the 1/2 cup of water using a whisk until all lumps are gone. Heat a skillet with some butter. Pour 1/4 of the batter into the hot buttered skillet (as if you are making crepes or pancakes, it does not take long so keep an eye on it). Allow the tortilla to "fry," when the edges are starting to brown, flip the tortilla, and cook for an additional 30 seconds. Do this for 4 tortillas.
Once done, let it cool a minute, then break them up into

"chips." Either salt them or sprinkle with cinnamon and sugar.

Makes 4 servings.

Grain Free Breads

Irish Soda Bread

This is a classic bread, enjoyed as a treat on St. Patrick's Day, but can also be enjoyed anytime as a grain free bread.

What You'll Need:

1 1/2 cups of rice flour (white)
1 cup of buttermilk
1/2 cup of tapioca flour
1/2 cup of sugar (granulated)
1 egg
1 teaspoon of baking soda
1 teaspoon of baking powder
1 teaspoon of salt

How to Make It:

Prep: Preheat the oven to 350 degrees Fahrenheit. Spray a 9 inch round pan with cooking spray.

In a bowl, combine the 1 1/2 cups of white rice flour, 1/2

cup of tapioca flour, 1/2 cup of granulated sugar, with the teaspoons of baking soda, baking powder, and salt. In a separate bowl, combine the cup of buttermilk and egg with a whisk. Pour into the center of the dry ingredients and stir until moistened. Batter may be lumpy. Pour into the prepared pan and bake for a little over an hour. Cake is done when a toothpick inserted in the middle comes out clean. Cool for 10 minutes, set pan on 2 knives or on a wire rack. Remove from pan and store wrapped in foil or plastic. Bread is best if it sits for a day before serving.

Makes 6 to 8 servings.

Corn Bread

Bake a pan of cornbread to go with a pot of beans or a bowl of chili.

What You'll Need:

2 eggs (lightly beaten)
1 1/2 cups of water (room temperature)
1 1/2 cup of cornmeal (fine)
1 cup of millet flour
1 cup of rice flour
1/4 cup of sugar (granulated)
1/4 cup of canola oil
1 tablespoon of baking powder
1 teaspoon of salt

How to Make It:

Prep: Preheat the oven to 350 degrees Fahrenheit. Spray a 9x9 inch baking pan with cooking spray.

In a bowl, combine the 2 lightly beaten eggs with the 1 1/2 cups of room temperature water and the 1/4 cup of canola oil with a whisk. In a separate bowl, combine the 1 1/2 cups of fine cornmeal, 1 cup of millet flour, 1 cup of rice flour, 1/4 cup of granulated sugar, tablespoon of baking powder, and the teaspoon of salt. Pour the liquid into the center of the dry ingredients and stir until just moistened. It may be slightly lumpy. Pour into the prepared 9x9 inch baking dish and bake for about 20 minutes, until the top turns golden and springy.

Makes 12 servings.

Herbed Parmesan Bread

This delicious herbed bread goes well with steamed vegetables and meat dishes.

What You'll Need:

2 1/2 cups of almond flour
1 cup of Parmesan cheese (grated)
3/4 cup of cottage cheese (large curd)
1/2 cup of water
2 eggs
3 tablespoons of butter (melted)
1 teaspoon of garlic (minced)
1/2 teaspoon of basil (dried)
1/2 teaspoon of baking soda
1/2 teaspoon of salt
1/3 teaspoon of oregano (dried)

1/3 teaspoon of thyme (dried)

How to Make It:

Prep: Preheat the oven to 325 degrees Fahrenheit. Spray 2 regular sized loaf pans with cooking spray.

Combine the 2 1/2 cups of almond flour with the cup of grated Parmesan cheese, 1/2 teaspoons of dried basil, baking soda, salt, 1/3 teaspoons of dried oregano, and dried thyme. Place the 3/4 cup of large curd cottage cheese, 1/2 cup of water, 2 eggs, 3 tablespoons of melted butter, and teaspoon of minced garlic into a food processor or blender. Blend until smooth. Add to the dry ingredients bowl and combine with a spoon. Divide the dough into 2 and place into the 2 loaf pans. Bake for just under an hour, when the top is golden brown.

Makes 2 loaves.

Banana Bread

This could be in the dessert section too, because it is that good.

What You'll Need:

3 cups of almond flour
1 cup of walnuts (chopped fine)
1/4 cup of honey
2 eggs (beaten)
2 bananas (ripe, peeled, mashed)
3 tablespoons of butter (melted)
3/4 teaspoon of baking soda
1/4 teaspoon of salt

How to Make It:

Prep: Preheat oven to 300 degrees Fahrenheit. Spray 2 regular sized loaf pans.

In a bowl, combine the 1/4 cup of honey, 2 beaten eggs, 2 ripe, peeled and mashed bananas, and 3 tablespoons of melted butter. In a separate bowl, combine the 3 cups of almond flour with the 3/4 teaspoon of baking soda, and 1/4 teaspoon of salt. Add the dry ingredients to the batter and mix. Stir in the cup of fine chopped walnuts. Divide equally between the two loaf pans. Bake for 50 minutes. Cool completely before serving.

Makes 2 loaves.

Sandwich Bread

This bread is perfect for making sandwiches or toast.

What You'll Need:

1 cup of cashew butter (room temperature)
4 eggs (separate the whites from the yolks)
1/4 cup of almond milk
1/4 cup of coconut flour
1 tablespoon of honey
2 1/2 teaspoons of apple cider vinegar
1 teaspoon of baking soda
1/2 teaspoon of salt

How to Make It:

Prep: Preheat oven to 300 degrees Fahrenheit. Place a sheet of parchment paper at the bottom of an 8.5x4.5 inch loaf pan. (Glass pan works best) Lightly spray the sides with cooking spray.

In a bowl, use an electric mixer to combine the cup of room temperature cashew butter with 4 egg yolks. Mix in the 1/4 cups of almond milk, tablespoon of honey, and the 2 1/2 teaspoons of apple cider vinegar for about a minute. In a separate bowl, add the 4 egg whites and beat them until stiff peaks form. In yet another bowl, combine the 1/4 cup of coconut flour with the teaspoon of baking soda and 1/2 teaspoon of salt. Next, add the dry ingredients to the milk mixture and beat for about a minute. Add the egg whites and beat long enough until it mixes well.   Add the dough to the prepared loaf pan and bake until a toothpick inserted in the middle comes out clean for around 47 minutes, until the top turns a nice golden brown. Immediately loosen the sides with a knife and remove loaf from pan and place on a wire rack for cooling before it is served.

Makes around 12 servings.

Zucchini Bread

This delicious zucchini bread is very moist and completely wheat free.

What You'll Need:

1 1/2 cups of zucchini (mashed)
1 1/2 cups of almonds (ground)
3/4 cup of almond butter
1/4 cup of arrowroot flour
1 egg
5 tablespoons of maple syrup
2 tablespoons of coconut oil
1 1/2 teaspoons of cinnamon (ground)
1 teaspoon of nutmeg (ground)
1 teaspoon of vanilla extract
1 teaspoon of baking soda

How to Make It:

Preheat oven to 325 degrees Fahrenheit. Lightly spray a regular sized loaf pan with cooking spray.

In a bowl, combine the 1 1/2 cups of mashed zucchini, 3/4 cups of almond butter, egg, 5 tablespoons of maple syrup, 2 tablespoons of coconut oil, and the teaspoon of vanilla extract. In a separate bowl, combine the 1/4 cup of arrowroot flour with the 1 1/2 teaspoon of ground cinnamon, teaspoon of ground nutmeg, and the teaspoon of baking soda. Add the dry ingredients to the wet ingredients, mix well. Add the 1 1/2 cups of ground almonds. Pour into the prepared loaf pan. Bake for 50 minutes. Allow to cool before serving.

Makes 1 loaf of bread.

Grain Free Side Dish Recipes

Broccoli Quinoa Casserole

This is the perfect side dish to pair with chicken or beef.

What You'll Need:

1 bunch of broccoli (florets, chopped)
1 tomato (chopped)
1 1/3 cups of water
1 cup of quinoa
1 cup of celery (chopped)
1/2 cup of onion (chopped)
3 tablespoons of soy sauce

2 tablespoons of brown rice vinegar
1 tablespoon of sesame oil (hot pepper)
2 teaspoons of curry powder
1/2 teaspoon of garlic (minced)

How to Make It:

Prep: Preheat the oven to 350 degrees Fahrenheit.

Place a skillet on medium high heat. Add the cup of quinoa and stir until it turns a golden brown and pops. Add the quinoa to a regular sized casserole dish. Pour in the 1 1/3 cups of water. Place a large pot on the stove and turn to medium high. Drizzle the hot pepper sesame oil into the pan, then sauté the 1/2 cup of chopped onions, 2 teaspoons of curry powder with the 1/2 teaspoon of minced garlic. Combine in the pot with the chopped broccoli florets, chopped tomato, and the cup of chopped celery. Stir and cook for 3 minutes. Add the 3 tablespoons of soy sauce and the 2 tablespoons of brown rice vinegar. Stir to combine and heat through. Pour over the quinoa. Bake in the oven until the top starts to brown, about 45 minutes. Let sit for 10 minutes, then serve.

Makes 4 servings.

Savory Black Bean Salad

This delicious salad has the savory and spicy flavor of the southwest with delicious couscous and black beans.

What You'll Need:

8 scallions (chopped)
2 cans of black beans (drained, 15 oz. each)
1 1/4 cups of chicken broth
1 cup of couscous (uncooked)
1 cup of corn (frozen, then thawed)
1/2 cup of bell pepper (red, seeded and chopped)
1/4 cup of cilantro (fresh, chopped)
3 tablespoons of olive oil (extra virgin)
2 tablespoons of lime juice
1 teaspoon of apple cider vinegar
1/2 teaspoon of cumin (ground)
salt and pepper

How to Make It:

Pour the 1 1/4 cups of chicken broth into a large saucepan and turn heat to high to bring to a boil. Add the cup of uncooked couscous and place a lid on the saucepan. Turn off heat and move pan off the burner for 5 minutes. Using a whisk, combine the 3 tablespoons of extra virgin olive oil, 2 tablespoons of lime juice, teaspoon of apple cider vinegar, with the 1/2 teaspoon of ground cumin in a bowl. Toss in the 8 chopped scallions, 2 cans of drained black beans, cup of thawed corn, 1/2 cup of chopped red bell pepper, and the 1/4 cup of fresh chopped cilantro. Next, using a fork, fluff the couscous and toss into the vegetables. Add salt and pepper to taste. Serve and enjoy.

Makes 8 servings.

Shrimp Soup

This soup makes a great lunch or a filling supper.

What You'll Need:

3/4 pound of shrimp (fresh, peeled, deveined)
3 cups of vegetable juice
1 bottle of clam juice (8 oz.)
1/2 cup of water
1/2 cup of long-grain white rice (uncooked)
1/2 cup of bell pepper (green, chopped)
1/4 cup of scallions (sliced)
1 bay leaf
1 tablespoon of butter
1/2 teaspoon of garlic (minced)
1/2 teaspoon of salt
1/4 teaspoon of thyme (dried)
1/4 teaspoon of basil (dried)
1/4 teaspoon of red pepper flakes
hot pepper sauce

How to Make It:

Place a large saucepan on stove and turn to medium heat. Add the tablespoon of butter and when it melts, add the 1/2 cup of chopped green bell pepper, 1/4 cup of sliced scallions, and the 1/2 teaspoon of minced garlic and sauté. Add the 3 cups of vegetable juice, bottle of clam juice, and the 1/2 cup of water and stir. Sprinkle in the 1/2 teaspoon of salt, 1/4 teaspoons of dried thyme, basil, and red pepper flakes. Add the bay leaf. Add the uncooked 1/2 cup of long-grain white rice. Turn to high until it boils, then turn to low to simmer, with cover, for 15 minutes, or until the rice is tender. Add the shrimp and cook for an additional 5 minutes. Remove and discard the bay leaf. Season with dashes of hot pepper sauce.

Makes 4 servings.

Mushroom Broccoli Tofu Quinoa

This is a hearty side dish but can double as a main dish because it is packed full of protein. It is perfect for vegetarians.

What You'll Need:

1 1/4 cups of vegetable broth (divided)
1 cup of spinach (chopped fresh)
1/2 cup of quinoa (uncooked)
1/2 cup of broccoli florets
1/2 cup of tofu (firm diced)
1/4 cup of mushrooms (sliced)
2 teaspoons of olive oil
2 teaspoons of garlic (minced)

How to Make It:

Pour the cup of vegetable broth into a saucepan and turn stove to high to bring to a boil. Add the 1/2 cup of uncooked quinoa, stir, reduce heat to low, cover with a lid and simmer for 20 minutes. Meanwhile, drizzle the 2 teaspoons of olive oil in a skillet and turn heat to medium. Add the 1/2 cup of broccoli florets, 1/2 cup of firm diced tofu, and the 2 teaspoons of mince garlic. Combine and then cover, turn heat to low and let sit for

2 minutes while it steams. Add the cup of chopped fresh spinach, 1/4 cup of vegetable broth, and the 1/4 cup of sliced mushrooms and stir. Turn heat up to medium, cover and cook for three more minutes. Add the vegetables to the quinoa pot, stir, cover, and sit with stove off for another 10 minutes. Transfer to a serving bowl, serve, and enjoy.

Makes 4 servings.

California Black Beans

This is a nice side dish that tastes great cool or warm.

What You'll Need:

4 cups of salsa
2 avocados (cubed)
1 1/2 cups of corn (whole kernels)
1 can of black beans (drained, rinsed)
1 cup of water
1/2 cup of quinoa

How to Make It:

Pour the water into a saucepan and add the 1/2 cup of

quinoa. Turn the stove to high to bring to a boil. Turn heat to medium low while quinoa cooks, until the water is absorbed, may take about 10 to 15 minutes. Pour the 1 1/2 cups of whole kernel corn and the can of drained, rinsed black beans into a serving bowl, toss in the cooked quinoa. Served with generous portion of salsa and cubed avocados on top.

Makes 4 servings.

Stuffing

This is the perfect side dish to go with any meat, or even a vegetable meal.

What You'll Need:

1 pound of sage turkey sausage
2 turnips (peeled and cubed)
1 apple (peeled, cored, diced)
5 cups of button mushrooms (diced)
3 1/2 cups of sweet potatoes (peeled and cubed)
2 1/2 cups of celery (diced)
1 1/2 cups of onions (diced)
2 1/2 teaspoons of garlic (powder)
2 1/2 teaspoons of sage (powder)
2 teaspoons of salt
1 teaspoon of oregano (dried)
1 teaspoon of rosemary (dried)
1 teaspoons of thyme (dried)
1 teaspoon of turmeric
1 teaspoon of black pepper
Canola oil (for cooking)

How to Make It:

Prep: Preheat the oven to 375 degrees Fahrenheit.

Spray 2 baking sheets with cooking spray.

Place the 2 peeled and cubed turnips and the 3 1/2 cups of peeled and cubed sweet potatoes in a large bowl. Spray the turnips and sweet potatoes with cooking spray. In a small cup add the 2 1/2 teaspoons of garlic powder, 2 1/2 teaspoons of sage powder, 2 teaspoons of salt, 1 teaspoon of dried oregano,1 teaspoon of dried rosemary, 1 teaspoons of dried thyme, 1 teaspoon of turmeric, and the 1 teaspoon of black pepper and combine. Sprinkle the seasonings over the sweet potatoes and turnips and toss to evenly coat. Spread the turnips and sweet potatoes out on the 2 baking sheets and place in the oven for an hour, turning every 15 minutes.

Meanwhile, add a little canola oil and cook the turkey sage sausage in a skillet until well done and brown. Add more canola oil if necessary, toss in the 2 1/2 cups of diced celery and the 1 1/2 cups of diced onions and sauté. Add the 5 cups of diced button mushrooms and the peeled, cored and diced apple, cook until they soften. Sprinkle extra seasonings over the sausage mixture if desired. Combine with the turnips and sweet potatoes. Spray a large baking dish - or a large roasting pan with cooking spray. Pour the contents into the pan. Reduce oven temperature to 350 degrees Fahrenheit and cook for half an hour. Alternatively, refrigerate the stuffing up to a day before cooking and serving.

Makes 8 servings.

Kale Mango Salad

A delicious and refreshing side dish.

What You'll Need:

1 bunch of kale (remove stalks, coarsely chopped)
1 cup of mango (diced)
1/4 cup of olive oil (plus a drizzle, extra virgin)
2 1/4 tablespoons of pumpkin seeds (toasted)
2 tablespoons of lemon juice (divided)
2 teaspoons of honey
Salt and pepper

How to Make It:

First, place the coarsely chopped kale in a large bowl, add a tablespoon of lemon juice and a drizzle of extra virgin olive oil. With hands, work the salt and lemon juice into the leaves, about 2 1/2 minutes of rubbing. Set to the side. In a separate smaller bowl, combine the remaining tablespoon of lemon juice with the 2 teaspoons of honey and several shakes of pepper. Add the 1/4 cup of extra virgin olive oil and continue whisking until it is well combined. Place the kale in 4 salad plates; divide the dice mango and pumpkin seeds. Drizzle the dressing over the salad and enjoy.

Makes 4 servings.

Grain Free Main Dish Recipes

Parmesan Mushrooms Quinoa

This dish is simply too hearty to be a side dish, it is a very tasty Italian style dish.

What You'll Need:

1 package of button mushrooms (8 ounces, chopped)
3 cups of chicken broth
1 1/2 cups of quinoa (rinsed)
1/2 cup of onions (chopped)
1/3 cup of Parmesan cheese (grated)
1 tablespoon of olive oil
1 tablespoon of butter
1/2 teaspoon of garlic (minced)

How to Make It:

Drizzle the tablespoon of olive oil into a skillet and turn heat to medium. Add the package of chopped mushrooms, 1/2 cup of chopped onions, and the 1/2 teaspoon of minced garlic and cook for five minutes, until well browned. Remove from heat. Add the tablespoon of butter to a saucepan and turn heat to medium high. Pour in the 1 1/2 cups of rinsed quinoa and brown, a couple of minutes. Add the 3 cups of chicken broth and turn to high until it boils, then reduce to simmer, for about ten minutes. Add the sautéed mushrooms, garlic, and onions and stir for 2 more minutes. Serve with Parmesan cheese sprinkled on top.

Makes 6 servings.

Meaty Red Beans and Rice

This dish is so good and the leftovers are even better.

What You'll Need:

1 pound of ground beef (lean)
1/2 pound of turkey kielbasa sausage (cut into bite sized chunks)
1 can of kidney beans (drained)
1 cup of pinto beans (canned, rinsed)
1 cup of vegetarian baked beans
3 1/4 cups of rice (white, uncooked)
1/4 cup of onion (minced)
1/2 teaspoon of cayenne pepper (ground)
canola oil

How to Make It:

Cook the 3 1/4 cups of rice according to package directions. Pour a little canola oil in a skillet and heat to medium high. Cook the 1/2 pound of turkey kielbasa sausage for about 7 minutes, stirring often to lightly brown on all sides. Sprinkle the 1/2 teaspoon of ground cayenne pepper. Put the turkey kielbasa sausage into the pot of rice. Add a little extra canola oil to the skillet if necessary, turn to medium high heat, and cook the pound of lean ground beef until browned. Add the pot of rice and sausage, add the 1/4 cup of minced onion, and continue to cook for another five minutes. Add the can of drained kidney beans, cup of caned, rinsed pinto beans and the cup of vegetarian baked beans, turn to simmer to heat through, stirring often. Add water if necessary to keep from sticking. Ready to serve when hot.

Makes 8 servings.

Fried Rice

This is a delicious main dish, hearty and filling, goes well with steamed vegetables or a salad.

What You'll Need:

1 package of green peas (frozen, 10 oz.)
1/2 pound of ground beef (lean)
2 scallions (chopped)
1 1/3 cups of rice (white, uncooked)
1 2/3 cups of water
1/8 cup of soy sauce
3 eggs (lightly beaten)
3 teaspoons of canola oil (divided)
1/4 teaspoon of salt
1/8 teaspoon of black pepper

How to Make It:

Add the 1 2/3 cups of water to a sauce pan and turn on high to bring to a boil. Add the 1 1/3 cups of white uncooked rice. Reduce the heat to low, stir, and cover. Simmer for 20 minutes. Crack the 3 eggs into a bowl and lightly beat. Add the 1/4 teaspoon of salt and 1/8 teaspoon of black pepper. Drizzle 1 teaspoon of canola oil in a large skillet and heat to medium high. Add the eggs, allowing them to cook evenly, stirring. Put in a bowl and set to the side. Cook the 1/2 pound of lean ground beef in the skillet until well browned. Drain the grease and put into another bowl. Drizzle the remaining 2 teaspoons of canola oil into the skillet and add the cooked rice. Stir the rice to fluff it. Add the cooked ground beef along with the cooked eggs, chopped scallions, and the 1/8 cup of soy sauce. Heat through, several minutes and serve hot.

Makes 4 servings.

Jambalaya

If you love the spiciness of Cajun food, you will love this Jambalaya dish.

What You'll Need:

2 chicken breasts (boneless, skinless, cut into bite sized chunks)
1/2 pound of turkey kielbasa sausage (diced)
4 cups of chicken stock
2 cups of rice (white uncooked)
1/2 cup of onion (diced)
1/2 cup of bell pepper (green, diced)
1/2 cup of celery (diced)
3 bay leaves
2 tablespoons of garlic (chopped)
2 teaspoons of Worcestershire sauce
2 teaspoons of olive oil
1 teaspoon of hot pepper sauce
1/2 teaspoon of onion powder
1/4 teaspoon of cayenne pepper
salt and pepper

How to Make It:

Drizzle the 2 teaspoons of olive oil in a large pot and

turn stove to medium high heat. Add the chunked chicken breasts and diced turkey kielbasa sausage and cook until done, several minutes. Add the 1/2 cup of diced onion, 1/2 cup of diced green bell pepper, 1/2 cup of diced celery, and the 2 tablespoons of chopped garlic and sauté for another five minutes. Add the 1/2 teaspoon of onion powder, 1/4 teaspoon of cayenne pepper, and dashes of salt and pepper and stir. Pour in the 2 cups of white uncooked rice and the 4 cups of chicken stock and stir. Add the 3 bay leaves and turn the heat to high to bring to a boil. Cover, reduce heat to simmer until the rice is tender, for about 20 minutes. Add the 2 teaspoons of Worcestershire sauce and the teaspoon of hot pepper sauce, toss and serve.

Makes 6 servings.

Stuffed Cabbage

This is a wonderfully filling delicious meal, the stick to your ribs kind.

What You'll Need:

1 pound of ground beef (lean)
1 head of cabbage
1 can of tomato juice (12 oz.)
1 cup of rice (cooked)
1 egg
1 tablespoon of vinegar
1 tablespoons of sugar (granulated)
garlic powder
water

How to Make It:
Rinse head of cabbage, peel off first outer layer of leaves and place into a large pot, add water to cover and place on stove on high heat to bring to a boil. Continue to boil until the cabbage is soft, about 15 minutes. Carefully remove the core, leaving the leaves intact. Next, in a bowl, add the pout of lean ground beef and mix together with the cup of cooked rice, egg, and a couple of dashes of garlic powder. Mix with your hands, forming balls that fit in your hand. Pull a leaf from the

cabbage and roll around the ball of meat, completely encasing the meat. Continue to do this until all the meat is gone. Place any leftover cabbage leaves in the bottom of a large pot. Place the cabbage rolls onto the leaves. Pour in the can of tomato juice, tablespoon of vinegar, tablespoon of granulated sugar, and add just enough water to cover the top of the cabbage rolls. Turn heat to medium low, cover the pot, and let simmer for an hour. Do not let the leaves burn.

Makes 8 servings.

Spicy Meatballs and Rice

This is a great main dish for beef lovers, with a Mexican twist.

What You'll Need:

1 pound of ground beef
1 can of tomato puree (14.25 oz.)
1 can of Mexican-style corn (11 oz., drained)
2 cups of water
1 cup of rice
1 cup of onions (minced and divided)
1 bay leaf
2 tablespoons of white vinegar
1 tablespoon of canola oil
2 tablespoons of parsley (dried divided)
1 tablespoon of brown sugar
2 1/2 teaspoons of oregano (dried, divided)
1 1/2 teaspoons of cumin
1 teaspoon of garlic (minced)
1/2 teaspoon of chili powder
salt and pepper

How to Make It:

In a bowl, add the pound of ground beef with the

tablespoon of dried parsley, 1 1/2 teaspoons of dried oregano, and salt to taste. Add the 2 cups of water to a saucepan and pour in the cup of rice. Turn heat to high to bring to a boil. Cover, reduce heat to simmer and cook for 20 minutes. Meanwhile, add the tablespoon of canola oil to a skillet and turn heat to medium. Add 1/2 cup of minced onions and 1/2 teaspoon of minced garlic and sauté. Add onions and garlic to the ground beef mixture. With hands, form two dozen meatballs. Add the meatballs to the already hot skillet, and brown all over. Next, drain most of the fat from the skillet. Leave enough to add the remaining 1/2 cup of minced onions and 1/2 teaspoon of minced garlic, and sauté this. Add the can of tomato puree, tablespoon of dried parsley, tablespoon of brown sugar, 1 teaspoon of dried oregano, 1 1/2 teaspoons of cumin, 1/2 teaspoon of chili powder, and salt and pepper, and stir. Add the bay leaf. Cook for about 20 minutes, until the liquid thickens. Continue to stir and add the meatballs, cooking an additional ten minutes. Make sure the meatballs are completely cooked. Stir in the can of Mexican-style corn and heat through. Serve over a bed of cooked rice.

Makes 4 servings.

Stuffed Peppers

A delicious main dish filled with seasoned beef.

What You'll Need:

6 bell peppers (green, cut the tops off and carefully remove the stem and seeds)
1 pound of ground beef (lean)
2 cans of tomato sauce (8 oz. each)
1 cup of water
1/2 cup of rice (white, long grain, uncooked)
1 tablespoon of Worcestershire sauce
1 teaspoon of Italian seasoning
1/4 teaspoon of garlic powder
1/4 teaspoon of onion powder
salt and pepper

How to Make It:

Prep: Preheat the oven to 350 degrees Fahrenheit.

Pour the cup of water into a saucepan, add the 1/2 cup of uncooked long grain white rice, and turn the heat to high. Bring to a boil, cover, reduce the heat to low and simmer for 20 minutes. Add the pound of lean ground beef to a skillet and cook on medium until brown . Next, place the 6 prepped green bell peppers in a baking dish, openings on top. In a bowl, add the cooked ground beef along with the cooked rice, 1 8 oz. can of tomato sauce, tablespoon of Worcestershire sauce, 1/4 teaspoon of garlic powder, 1/4 teaspoon of onion powder and salt and pepper. Divide and spoon into each green bell pepper. In a separate bowl, mix the remaining 8 oz. can of tomato sauce with the tablespoon of Italian seasoning. Drizzle the sauce over the tops of the green bell peppers. Bake for an hour, basting with the tomato sauce at least 4 times.

Makes 6 servings.

Salmon and Rice

This is a delicious and nutritious meal made with smoked salmon and tasty fried rice.

What You'll Need:

6 cups of water
3 cups of rice (uncooked, long grain, white)
4 oz. of smoked salmon (chopped)
2 eggs (beaten)
1 scallion (chopped)
3 tablespoons of canola oil (divided)
1/2 cup of English peas (frozen)
1/4 cup of onions (fine chopped)
salt and pepper

How to Make It:

Add the 6 cups of water to a large saucepan on the stove on high heat. Add the 3 cups of uncooked long grain white rice and bring to a boil. Cover, reduce heat to low, and simmer until the rice is tender, about 20 minutes. Next, pour 2 tablespoons of canola oil into a skillet on medium heat. Add the 2 beaten eggs and scramble. Place eggs in a small bowl and set aside. Add the remaining tablespoon of canola oil to the skillet keep heat on medium. Add the chopped scallion and the 1/4 cup of fine chopped onions and sauté. Add the 4 oz. of chopped smoked salmon, cooked rice, scrambled eggs, and the 1/2 cup of frozen English peas and combine well. Season with salt, pepper, and heat through.

Makes 6 servings.

Seafood Gumbo

A hearty meal of seafood gumbo tastes great and is very filling if served over a bed of rice.

What You'll Need:

1 pound of shrimp (peeled, deveined, shelled)
7 cups of vegetable stock
2 cups of celery (chopped)
2 cups of onion (chopped)
2 cups of oysters (shucked)
2 cups of bell pepper (chopped, 1 red and 1 green)
1 1/2 cups of tomato sauce
1 cup of crabmeat
3/4 cup of canola oil
1 bay leaf
3 tablespoons of cornstarch
2 teaspoons of hot pepper sauce
1 1/2 teaspoons of paprika
1 teaspoon of garlic (minced)
1 teaspoon of salt
1/2 teaspoon of thyme (dried)
1/2 teaspoon of oregano (dried)
1/2 teaspoon of cayenne pepper (ground)
1/2 teaspoon of white pepper (ground)
1/2 teaspoon of black pepper (ground)

How to Make It:

In a small cup, combine the 1 1/2 teaspoons of paprika, teaspoon of salt, 1/2 teaspoons of dried, thyme, dried oregano, ground cayenne pepper, ground white pepper, and ground black pepper. Add the bay leaf. Set aside. Place a heavy large pot over medium high heat; add the 3/4 cup of canola oil. Stir in the 2 cups of chopped celery, 2 cups of chopped onion, 2 cups of chopped red and green bell peppers. Turn the heat to high, stirring often, add the 3 tablespoons of cornstarch, 2 teaspoons of hot pepper sauce, teaspoon of minced garlic, and the small cup of herbs, and stir for 5 minutes. Add the 1 1/2 cups of tomato sauce and keep stirring while turning the heat to high. Pour in the 7 cups of vegetable stock and bring to a boil. Turn heat to low and simmer for 60 minutes. Stir occasionally. Add the pound of peeled, deveined, and shelled shrimp, 2 cups of shucked oysters, and the cup of crabmeat, cover and cook for 5 minutes. Turn the burner off and allow it to stand for ten more minutes. Serve hot.

Makes 8 servings.

Chicken Salad

This is a very simple, yet filling recipe for chicken salad, excellent for lunch or supper.

What You'll Need:

1 apple (cored, peeled, diced)
1 chicken breast (boneless, skinless, cooked, shredded)
1 cup of pecans (chopped)
2/3 cup of raisins
1/4 cup of celery (chopped)
1/4 cup of onions (chopped)
3 tablespoons of mayonnaise
1 tablespoon of dill pickle relish
salt and pepper

How to Make It:

Combine the 3 tablespoons of mayonnaise with the tablespoon of dill pickle relish and dashes of salt and pepper, using a whisk. In a separate bowl, add the cored, peeled, and diced apple, shredded chicken breast, cup of chopped pecans, 2/3 cup of raisins, 1/4 cup of chopped celery, and 1/4 chopped onions and toss to combine. Pour the mayonnaise dressing over it and toss to coat evenly. Chill for at least half an hour before serving. Serve with lettuce, bread, or crackers.

Makes 6 servings.

Chicken Curry

Chicken curry is a favorite among many and completely grain free.

What You'll Need:

2 pounds of chicken breasts (boneless, skinless, chunked)
1 1/2 cup of onions (chopped)
1/4 cup of olive oil
1 bay leaf
3 tablespoons of curry powder
1 tablespoon of lemon juice
1 tablespoon of tomato paste
1 teaspoon of garlic (minced)
1 teaspoon of cinnamon (ground)
1 teaspoon of paprika
1/2 teaspoon of cayenne pepper
1/2 teaspoon of sugar (granulated)
1/4 teaspoon of ginger (ground)
salt
water

How to Make It:

Pour the 1/4 cup of olive oil in a skillet and turn to

medium high heat. Add the 1 1/2 cup of chopped onions and sauté. Stir in the teaspoon of ground cinnamon and add the bay leaf. Stir in the 3 tablespoons of curry powder, teaspoon of minced garlic, teaspoon of paprika, 1/2 teaspoon of granulated sugar, 1/4 teaspoon of ground ginger, and a few dashes of salt. Cook for a couple of minutes, until the mixture thickens. Stir in the 2 pounds of boneless, skinless, chunked chicken breasts and the tablespoon of tomato paste. Add water until all the chicken is completely covered. Stir and cook on medium low for 20 minutes. Add the tablespoons of lemon juice and the 1/2 teaspoon of cayenne pepper before serving.

Makes 6 servings.

Californian Chicken Soup

This is a delicious soup with avocados, Monterey Jack cheese, and a lot of flavor to make you think of California.

What You'll Need:

2 cans of green chili peppers (4.5 oz. each, drained, diced)
1 can of garbanzo beans (15 oz., drained)
2 chipotle peppers in adobo sauce (minced)
1 avocado (peeled, pitted, sliced)
4 cups of chicken broth
2 cups of chicken (cooked and shredded)
1 cup of rice (white, cooked)
1 cup of Monterey Jack cheese (shredded)
1 teaspoon of oregano (dried)
salt and pepper

How to Make It:

Add the 4 cups of chicken broth to a large soup pot, turn to medium high and just before it boils, turn to low. Add the can of garbanzo beans, 2 minced chipotle peppers, 2 cups of cooked shredded chicken, cup of cooked white rice, and salt and pepper. Simmer on medium low for half an hour. If the soup is too thick, add more chicken broth. Serve by spooning into bowls and topping with a slice of avocado and some shredded Monterey cheese.

Makes 6 servings.

Beef Stew

An all-time favorite, beef stew is the ultimate in comfort foods.

What You'll Need:

2 pounds of beef stew
2 cups of water (divided)
1 1/2 cups of carrots (sliced)
1 1/2 cups of celery (chopped)
1/2 cup of onions (sliced)
1 bay leaf
2 tablespoons of canola oil
2 tablespoons of cornstarch
1 tablespoon of Worcestershire sauce
1 teaspoon of salt
1 teaspoon of sugar (granulated)
1/2 teaspoon of black pepper
1/2 teaspoon of paprika
1/2 teaspoon of garlic (minced)
Dash of allspice (ground)

How to Make It:

Add the 2 tablespoons of canola oil to a skillet and turn the heat to medium high. Add the 2 pounds of stew meat and brown all sides. Transfer the meat to a large pot and add the 1 3/4 cups of water, 1/2 cup of sliced onions, 1 tablespoon of Worcestershire sauce, teaspoon of salt, teaspoon of granulated sugar, 1/2 teaspoon of black pepper, 1/2 teaspoon of paprika, 1/2 teaspoon of minced garlic, and a dash of ground allspice and stir. Drop in the bay leaf, cover and reduce heat to low and simmer for 90 minutes. Remove and discard the bay leaf. Add the 1 1/2 cups of sliced carrots and the 1 1/2 cups of chopped celery, replace the cover and cook for another 40 minutes. Mix 1/4 cup of remaining water with the 2 tablespoons of cornstarch with a whisk. Pour into the stew, stir, and turn heat up to medium high. Stir and cook until it starts to boil, then turn it off and cool to serve.

Makes 6 servings.

Baked Salmon

Salmon is a very healthy food to eat giving the body a good supply of Omega 3 fatty acids. This recipe is a delicious means of giving the body what it needs to stay healthy.

What You'll Need:

4 salmon filets
1 can of tomatoes (chopped, drained, 14 oz.)
3/4 cup of onions (chopped)
2 1/2 tablespoons of olive oil (divided)
2 tablespoons of lemon juice
1 teaspoon of oregano (dried)
1 teaspoon of thyme (dried)
Salt and pepper

How to Make It:

Prep: Preheat oven to degrees Fahrenheit.

Lay the salmon out and drizzle with 1/2 tablespoon of olive oil and sprinkle with salt and pepper. In a bowl, combine the drained can of tomatoes, 3/4 cup of chopped onions, 2 tablespoons of lemon juice, 2 tablespoons of olive oil, teaspoon of dried oregano, and teaspoon of dried thyme. Use a baking sheet that will hold all four fillets, place a sheet of foil down in the bottom, leave it loose. Lay each salmon fillet down on the foil, on the side that was oiled, salted and peppered. Next, spoon the seasoned tomatoes over the salmon, evenly covering all fillets. Take another sheet of foil and place over the top of the fillets, and fold over the edges, rolling them up to make a tight seal, sealing all the fillets inside a large foil "packet." Bake for under 30 minutes, until the salmon is cooked.

Makes 4 servings.

Dutch Oven Chili

This chili recipe certainly creates a pot full of comfort food you will want to eat on for a couple of days, because it is that good.

What You'll Need:

1 pound of ground beef (lean)
2 cups of water
1 can of tomatoes (28 oz., crushed)
1 can of black beans (15.5 oz., drained, rinsed)
1 can of kidney beans (15.5 oz., drained, rinsed)
1 can of pinto beans (15.5 oz., drained, rinsed)
1 cup of onions (diced)
1 cup of bell peppers (red, diced)
1/2 cup of carrots (diced)
1 chipotle chili in adobo sauce (seeded, minced)
1 tablespoon of olive oil
2 teaspoons of adobo sauce
2 teaspoons of cumin (ground)
1/2 teaspoons of oregano (dried)
salt and pepper

How to Make It:

Place a Dutch oven on medium heat. Drizzle the

tablespoon of olive oil in the bottom then add the 1 cup of diced onions, 1 cup of diced red bell pepper, and 1/2 cup of diced carrots. Cover the pot, cook, and stir occasionally for 10 minutes or until all the vegetables are tender. Add the 2 teaspoons of ground cumin, and stir for 60 seconds. Add the ground beef, making it crumble as it browns over high heat. Add the 2 cups of water, can of crushed tomatoes, minced chipotle chili pepper, 2 teaspoons of adobo sauce, 1/2 teaspoon of dried oregano, and dashes of salt and pepper. Lay the lid crossways, so it's not completely covered and turn the heat down to low, stirring occasionally for a half an hour. Add the cans of black, kidney and pinto beans, keep the lid the same, stirring once in a while, and cook for another 20 minutes. Salt and pepper to taste.

Makes 8 servings.

5 Day Meal Plan

These are just suggestions of using some of the recipes within this book on a daily basis. You need to include vegetables and fruit and nuts in your diet as well. Always fix extra vegetables and or a salad with supper.

Day 1

Breakfast - Vanilla Yogurt with Fruit Salad

Snack - Nuts

Lunch - Grain free bread sandwich

Snack - Tortilla chips and salsa

Supper - Beef Stew

Dessert - Banana Date Cookies

Day 2

Breakfast - Oven Omelet

Snack - Piece of fruit

Lunch - Shrimp Soup

Snack - nuts

Supper - Seafood Gumbo

Dessert - Classic No Bake Cookies

Day 3

Breakfast - Sweet Potato Breakfast Casserole

Snack - nuts

Lunch - Kale Mango Salad

Snack - piece of fruit

Supper - Stuffed Peppers

Dessert - Ginger cookies

Day 4

Breakfast - Coffee Cake

Snack - piece of fruit

Lunch - Savory Black Bean Salad

Snack - nuts

Supper - Chicken Curry

Dessert - Oatmeal Chocolate Chip Raisin Cookies

Day 5

Breakfast - Breakfast Burrito

Snack - Piece of Fruit

Lunch - Chili and Corn bread

Snack - nuts

Supper - Baked Salmon

Dessert - Raisin Nut Cake

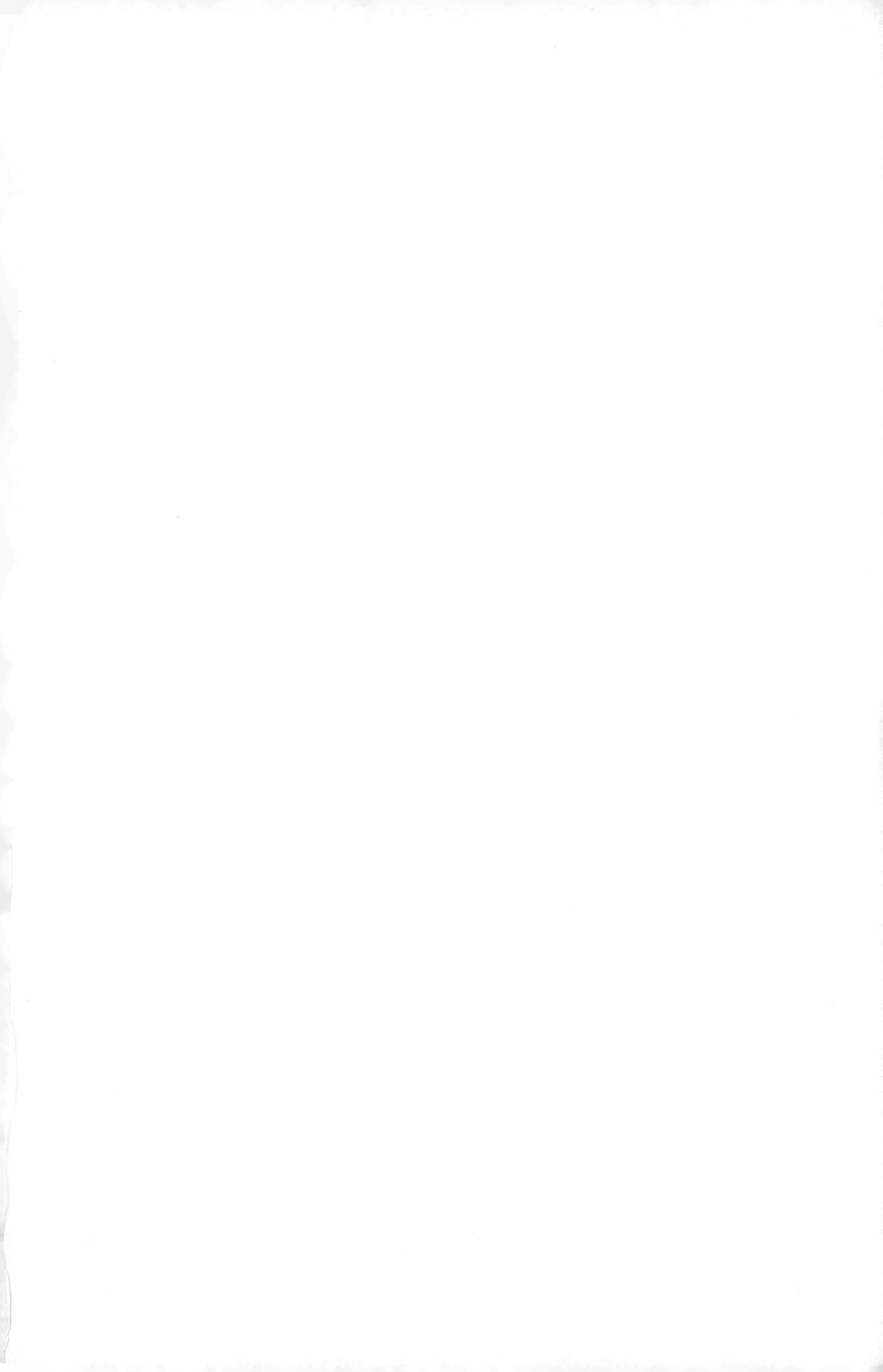

www.ingramcontent.com/pod-product-compliance
Ingram Content Group UK Ltd.
Pitfield, Milton Keynes, MK11 3LW, UK
UKHW020652130126
10066UKWH00028B/453